Making Sense of a Primary Care-Led Health Service

Edited by

PETER LITTLEJOHNS

Director of the Health Care Evaluation Unit
St George's Hospital Medical School

and

CHRISTINA VICTOR

Senior Lecturer in Health Services Research
St George's Hospital Medical School

Foreword by

ROGER JONES

Wolfson Professor of General Practice
UMDS (Guy's and St Thomas')

Radcliffe Medical Press
Oxford and New York

© 1996 Peter Littlejohns and Christina Victor

Radcliffe Medical Press Ltd
18 Marcham Road, Abingdon, Oxon OX14 1AA, UK

Radcliffe Medical Press, Inc.
141 Fifth Avenue, New York, NY 10010, USA

British Library Cataloguing in Publication Data

A catalogue record for this book is available from the British Library.

ISBN 1 85775 048 9

Library of Congress Cataloging-in-Publication Data is available.

Typeset by Advance Typesetting Ltd, Oxon
Printed and bound by Redwood Books, Trowbridge, Wiltshire

Contents

List of contributors

Dr Ralph Burton
Senior Lecturer in General Practice
St George's Hospital Medical School
Cranmer Terrace
Tooting
London SW17 0RE

Dr Tim Crayford
Lecturer in Public Health
King's College Hospital and Dental School
Bessemer Road
London SE5 9PJ

Dr Howard Freeman
General Practitioner
12 Durham Road
West Wimbledon
London SW20 0TW

Dr Siân Griffiths
Director of Public Health and Health Policy
Oxfordshire Health Authority
Old Road
Headington
Oxford OX3 7LG

Dr Andrew Harris
Honorary Lecturer in General Practice and Senior Registrar in Public Health
King's College Hospital Medical School
Bancroft Unit
Tower Hamlets Health Care Trust
London E1 4DG

Dr Peter Littlejohns
Director of the Health Care Evaluation Unit
St George's Hospital Medical School
Cranmer Terrace
Tooting
London SW17 0RE

Dr Azeem Majeed
Lecturer in Public Health Medicine
Department of Public Health Sciences
St George's Hospital Medical School
Cranmer Terrace
Tooting
London SW17 0RE

Dr Jonathan McWilliam
Consultant in Public Health
Oxfordshire Health Authority
Old Road
Headington
Oxford OX3 7LG

Dr John Shanks
Consultant in Public Health Medicine
Lambeth, Southwark and Lewisham Health Authority
1 Lower Marsh
London SE1 7NT

Dr Christina Victor
Senior Lecturer in Health Services Research
Department of Public Health Sciences
St George's Hospital Medical School
Cranmer Terrace
Tooting
London SW17 0RE

Dr Andrew Willis
Chairman
The National Association of Commissioning General Practitioners
19 Thorburn Road
Northampton
NN3 3DA

Foreword

The central research and development committee of the NHS R&D programme recognized the importance of the interface between primary and secondary care four years ago and commissioned an extensive programme of research on a number of priority topics. Many of these topics are reflected in the subjects and themes of this timely book, which deals with a number of important questions for policy, management and research in the health service. The editors and authors have provided valuable landmarks in a key area of change that is still being mapped.

Re-appraisal and re-configuration of health services is taking place across the world and shifts in the interface between primary and secondary care are particularly apparent in North America and North Eastern Europe. They are based at least partly on the recognition of the value of a strong primary care service, a belief reflected in the structures of emerging health care systems in many non-European countries. Whilst the imperatives of national economies and health care policies are powerful forces for change, it is also important to recognize the equally potent effects on the interface of changes in medical practice, advances in information technology, drug therapy, near-patient diagnostics and, not least, a growing sense of confidence and maturity in general practice, which long predated the creation of the internal market and EL(94)79.

We are now spectators of a fascinating range of natural experiments in health policy taking place around the globe, in relation to registration and capitation systems, health maintenance organizations, changes in traditional roles, the mix of skills required for health care delivery and innovations in funding arrangements for health care. One experiment being watched with a high degree of interest is, of course, the purchaser–provider arrangements developed within the NHS, and the increasing role played by primary care professionals in commissioning services.

As the interface shifts and becomes blurred, so the nature and shape of primary care itself also alters and the roles and responsibilities of those working in it change. Challenging and exciting times lie ahead, but we also face considerable problems in primary care, not least those of low morale and difficulties in recruiting high-quality graduates and registrars to general practice. Despite their best intentions, many general practitioners can find no slack in the system and are concerned that the demands being placed on primary care are not underpinned by a commensurate shift of resources. Indeed, moving the focus of care from the hospital to the community may not necessarily be cheaper and the systematic care of chronic disease may turn out to be more expensive than unstructured, sporadic care.

These shifts in the focus of clinical care are mirrored by changing perceptions of the community as an appropriate setting for teaching and research. The Winyard Report emphasized the importance of creating a mechanism to provide adequate funding for general practitioners involved in undergraduate education, while the Culyer Report similarly emphasized the need to identify a funding stream to provide a research and development infrastructure for research in primary care and community settings. This is also echoed in the work of the NHS R&D strategy and strategic thinking in the Medical Research Council.

The creation of an evaluative culture in general practice, with a strengthened research and development infrastructure linked to enhanced academic training opportunities, the promotion of evidence-based practice and the creation of strong new alliances between clinical and academic general practice should contribute to the provision of the new skills, confidence and resources required to deliver a first class primary care service in the UK. The editors and authors of this book have done a superb job in charting the way ahead.

Roger Jones
Wolfson Professor of General Practice
UMDS (Guy's and St Thomas')

April 1996

Introduction

Peter Littlejohns

> *Good quality primary care is being recognized throughout the world as the basis of a cost-effective health service. In the UK this approach has been adopted by the government with the emphasis on the National Health Service becoming a 'primary care-led service'. Rather than being considered merely a gatekeeper to expensive secondary care, the provision of health care by general practitioners, nurses and others is now recognized in its own right. Furthermore as general practitioners become more involved in the commissioning and purchasing of secondary care, the balance of the management of the health service is shifting away from hospital based consultants and general managers to general practitioners. However the speed of this policy implementation and the lack of systematic evaluation has left many clinicians and managers, both sides of the primary/secondary care interface, unsure of what it really means. What are the long-term implications?*

What is a primary care-led health service?

In essence a primary care-led health service will require general practitioners to take a public as well as personal health perspective. They will have to work within limited resources allocated on the basis of need, prioritize the services they purchase and manage large business consortia. All this at the same time as providing an expanded primary care service.

There are numerous books, many from this publishing house, that deal specifically with the myriad of new skills and knowledge required by general practitioners and their teams. This book, however, deals with the overall concept of the policy and its implementation through the eyes of general practitioners and public health physicians who actually have to make it work on a day-to-day basis. Chapter two deals with the origins of the policy and identifies its key features and how it will affect primary care workers.

Resourcing the policy

It has been argued that for the primary care-led policy to work, a shift in the balance of resources away from hospitals to the community is required. This call takes place at a time when the demand for secondary care shows no sign of diminishing. Emergency admissions are increasing to the extent that, once again, stories of patients waiting for hours on trolleys in hospital corridors result in questions on the floor of the House of Commons. Other health policies on manpower, clinical involvement in audit and management, changing training and postgraduate education requirements and new clinical practices are resulting in the view that workloads will increase, not decrease, in hospitals. Consultant morale is low.

> *There is widespread concern amongst physicians that increasing pressure to take on ever more work is impeding their ability to practise the high standards of medicine to which they aspire. Uncertainty, frustration and even despondency are beginning to threaten the sense of commitment to the NHS of many physicians in adult and paediatric practice. I constantly bring to the attention of the Department of Health and the NHS Executive the damage that this is causing to the quality and standard of care we provide …*

> Letter to members of Royal College of Physicians, 14th December 1995, from the president Professor Sir Leslie Turnberg.

It is unlikely in this climate that a major change in the balance of resources, resulting in a withdrawal of funds from hospitals, will be politically acceptable. The argument that good primary care leads to a reduction in the use of secondary care applies at a macro level, and possibly, given time, at a micro level. It does not however occur quickly, and certainly not until the requisite community services are in place; a lesson currently being learnt by carers of mentally ill patients who have been discharged from secondary services to a community ill equipped to cope. So in the short-term, unless the health service receives a massive injection of new funding, implementation of the primary care-led policy will mean a redistribution of more or less current resources.

Information

Markets can only thrive on information and a 'health market' is no exception. Indeed the value of reliable, relevant and rapid information is reinforced by it being raised in every chapter of this book. Two key areas warrant chapters in their own right: information for needs assessment and for monitoring the service's performance.

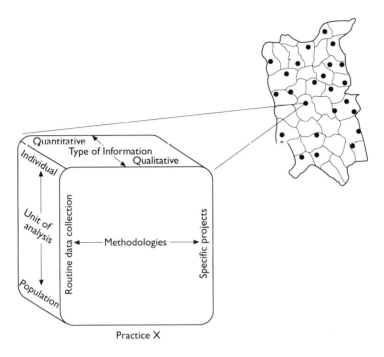

Figure 1.1   Practice-based needs assessment: three dimensions to consider.

Assessing needs: patients, population ... or practice?

With finite resources, needs assessment is as much about prioritizing the services a practice can provide as seeking out undiscovered need. On the basis that you are raising expectations that cannot be realized, the value of needs assessment has been questioned and a process of marginal analysis offered as an alternative.[1] Many practices are already wary and view needs assessment as a way of securing more resources by challenging assumptions about resource allocation. Needs assessment, like many of the other elements of the new thinking, has an important role: conceptually it is the key to a rational basis for equitable health care provision. However it does not necessarily have to dominate the process. Practices will need to decide on which method and how much resource they wish to invest (Figure 1.1). Health authorities will have to fit the pieces together and speculate on the missing ones. In chapter three John Shanks and Tim Crayford describe how routine databases and surveys can be used in conjunction with qualitative methods to create an overall picture.

Monitoring quality and performance

In chapter four Azeem Majeed describes how you can also use these sources of data to monitor the performance of general practitioner activities. However in a professionally-led service, quality initiatives should also reflect the ethos of that profession. In health care the classical ways have been through audit and education. In chapter seven Ralph Burton describes how this can be made to work in a contractual setting.

Purchasing health care – are markets obsolete?

The fundamental difference of the present arrangements in primary care compared to before the reforms is the influence that general practitioners have on the organization of secondary as well as primary care. The starting place for this revolution was the concept of general practitioners being responsible for budgets with which to purchase secondary services. In chapter five Howard Freeman describes the evolution of fundholding, its strengths in bringing about change, and argues that it still has much to offer.

However a number of commentators of the NHS reforms consider that the competition ethos is beginning to burn out. Successive Secretaries of State for Health, faced with the lack of competition in many parts of the country, the high managerial and transaction costs, the considerable opportunity costs for professionals and the unacceptability of 'market losers', are now emphasizing the need for co-ordination, collaboration and long-term contracting. If true, this would suggest that alliances between health authorities and general practitioners rather than competitive purchasing, may be the way forward.[2] In chapter six Andrew Willis proposes a model of how general practitioners can exert influence through commissioning.

Hospitals – who needs them?
What elements of care can be shifted out of hospital?

While the new role general practitioners have in planning overall services and commissioning secondary care is exciting, their main function remains the provision of health care directly to patients. Because the bulk of health care takes place in primary care with only a small proportion being referred to the secondary sector, minor changes in decision making can lead to massive changes in the use of hospitals. For example, an assessment of all patients with asthma in one group practice revealed that only about ten per cent had been referred to an outpatient clinic.[3] Linking this to the number of patients seen at the local asthma clinic revealed that if this was similar for other practices, then a 10% rise in the threshold for referring (i.e. each GP referring nine rather than ten patients) would halve the number of patients being seen at the hospital. This sort of simple calculation forms the basis of the thinking behind the policy in the first place. However the alternative is also possible, minor changes in global factors that affect a whole patient population can swamp a hospital service. The steeper the sides of the pyramid between the prevalence of the problem in primary compared to secondary care, the more unstable the situation. This may explain why we remain unclear over the reasons for the continuing increase in the number of acute medical admissions to hospitals. We postulate that the increase could be due to a number of factors, including:

- changing demography
- too rapid turn-round in hospital leading to re-admission
- reduced family support
- poor community services
- increasing morbidity
- more conditions amenable to treatment
- increased patient expectations
- better paramedic services
- market incentive to create emergency cases.

But we do not have the answer. It seems absurd in these days of evidence-based medicine that this most basic of questions, i.e. why are more people being admitted to hospital, remains resistant to a definitive answer. Moreover attempts to respond with various schemes have been fragmented and largely unevaluated. Surely a large multi-centre trial of the schemes to prevent inappropriate admission and speed discharge needs to be commissioned by the National Research and Development Initiative.

Understanding this phenomenon is crucial to the success of a primary care-led service, particularly as perceived by the public. While they may want their chronic disease managed locally, they do not want it to be at the expense of rapid emergency treatment whenever they or their family require it. Discussions over 'utilitarian' theories of resource allocation and risk management strategies will not stand up against *News at Ten* reporting yet another patient being diverted from hospital to hospital, by helicopter, because no bed is available. Furthermore, popular public affection remains closely linked to their hospital and specialty staff and a considerable educational task is required to convince them otherwise.[4]

Whatever the size of the shift to primary care, hospitals will continue to have a significant role in the future health service. In chapter eight Christina Victor addresses the ubiquitous problems of getting patients in and out of hospital with the minimum of inconvenience.

Who manages the new NHS?

April 1996 saw the demise of regional health authorities, family health services authorities and district health authorities and the birth of regional offices of the

NHS Executive, and new joint authorities. What are their role and how can they link with general practitioners? Siân Griffiths and Jonathan McWilliam present the principles as well as the likely difficulties in chapter nine.

New roles or new people?

To cope with the increasing responsibilities managerial staff are proliferating in general practices, changing the 'cottage industry' image to that of large organizations with multi-million pound revenues, managed by chief executives. However it is unlikely that this will lead to significant reductions in managerial workloads for general practitioners. The Royal College of General Practitioners is aware of this misconception and in their latest occasional paper[5] suggest that while practice managers can minimize the considerable increase in bureaucracy that a primary care-led service creates, ultimately key decisions have to be made by doctors and hence their involvement is crucial and time consuming. They emphasize that whatever the new roles for general practitioners, their most important one occurs during the face-to-face contact with patients. It is this role that needs to be maximized and is probably the element of British primary care that is likely to be the key to a cost-effective service. Therefore new organizational changes should seek to maximize this aspect of care rather than reduce it.

Much is said about the potential of changing the skill-mix in primary care, and increasing the involvement of nurses and professions allied to medicine to lessen the doctor's load. While there is no doubt that the quality of care can be improved by the use of other health care professionals, careful research can show that this does not necessarily reduce doctors' time or health service costs. For example, introducing a nurse practitioner into the management of patients with chronic obstructive lung disease improved the quality of life of patients and kept them alive longer, but increased the number of times a general practitioner saw them and increased the drugs bill.[6]

However there remain enough examples of successful re-organization of local services and altering skill-mix to make this an important component of a primary care-led service. Fundamental to these changes is the involvement of patients. Simple surveys of patients' expectations can provide the rationale for a complete rethink on how services have been traditionally provided, e.g. changing hearing aid provision from a consultant to audiologist-led service to increase effective uptake and reduce hospital waiting lists.[7]

General practitioners and public health physicians – a reversal of roles?

At the heart of the general practitioner purchasing debate is how successfully doctors can act as advocates for individual patients and whole populations at the same time. This latter practice has historically been the role of public health physicians who can advise on priorities without having to face individual patients on a day-to-day basis (and tell them that they are a low priority). Fundholding means that general practitioners will have to assume both roles. So far this has not needed to happen as funding has been generous. But as resource allocation moves from historical activity to a capitation basis, no practice will avoid having to face these decisions in the future. Advocates will argue that these decisions have always been made by (implicitly) selectively referring patients to hospital. But protagonists argue that this is very different to the explicit way that will be needed in the future. This is the real difference between purchasing and commissioning. Advocates of GPs only being involved in the latter hope to exert influence without having to be responsible for rationing. However it remains to be seen whether this influence can work. Professional advisory systems have been in place for many years without real influence. There is no doubt that the acquisition of budgets by GPs has increased the listening power of trusts. However it may be that while fundholding may be seen as the vehicle of change it may be less adroit at sustaining it over time. Already the prescribing savings being offered as an example of the success of fundholding in Oxford have been lost over time.[8]

Intriguingly in recent years as GPs have become more literate in needs assessment of their practice populations, seek to understand the cost-effectiveness of their interventions and evaluate their performance, they have acted more and more like public health physicians (without distancing themselves from their patients of course). At the same time public health physicians have become increasingly interested in individual patients. Where can we place patient X, with a severe debilitating disease, when the relatives can no longer cope? Why was there no intensive therapy unit bed for patient Y? Why cannot couple Z have NHS fertility treatment when a similar couple living a few miles away can?

This blending of roles is likely to increase as one of the results of the primary care-led service will be an increased understanding of each individual professional's contribution. This is equally happening with hospital consultants as they become involved in Health of the Nation programmes to prevent as well as treat disease. In the new health service it is becoming difficult to divorce one element of care from another. Politicians love pushing each new health policy as the answer to the health service problems. Over the last few years we have had: general management, resource management, purchaser and provider split, quality assurance, total quality management, clinical audit, clinical guidelines, evidence-based medicine and now a primary care-led health policy. Each was supposed to be a huge step forward, each less than realized its purported potential, but all reinforced the need for all professionals in the NHS to work closer together. Many of the policies over the last few years have been perceived to be divisive, but most have lost their teeth in the implementation. The primary care-led policy is probably the same as the others; we need to develop cautiously what is likely to be better without discarding what we already know is good.

Sustainability

Much of the initial drive to improve primary care services has been through the infusion of targeted 'pump-priming' finances to specific problem areas, e.g. the London Implementation Zone. Because there has been the political imperative to demonstrate rapid results, funding has been project-based in response to hastily produced action plans. Many of these plans seek to apply 'good practice' schemes developed elsewhere to their local problems, and have had to use non-recurring revenue. It is unlikely that this approach will provide a lasting solution because they ignore the underlying reasons for the problem in the first place. Slower but sustainable changes in primary care personnel and infra-structure associated with educational programmes are more likely to be effective.

Diversity

In describing the new primary care-led National Health Service in the *British Medical Journal*,[9] Professor Chris Ham suggests that we will have to learn to live with diversity. This book mirrors that prophesy. In bringing together a range of authors there is a multiplicity of views, beliefs and styles. In order not to dilute the impact, other than making some minor changes, the text has been left unchanged. What this reveals (whatever the viewpoint) is a passionate belief in the excellence of the National Health Service and the desire for primary care to make a major contribution. We do not attempt to provide all the answers, but we hope that by reading this book the reader will more fully understand the issues that need to be addressed if a primary care-led service is to realize its potential.

References

1   Cohen D. (1994) Marginal analysis in practice: an alternative to needs assessment for contracting health care. *British Medical Journal.* **309**: 781–5.

2   Bottomly V. (1995) *The New NHS: continuity and change.* Department of Health, London.

3   Littlejohns P, Ebrahim S, Anderson R. (1989) Treatment of adult asthma: is the diagnosis relevant? *Thorax.* **44**: 797–802.

4   Coulter A. (1995) Shifting the balance from secondary to primary care: needs investment and cultural change. *British Medical Journal.* **311**: 1447–8.

5   Royal College of General Practitioners. (1995) *The Nature of General Medical Practice.* Report from general practice number 27.

6   Littlejohns P, Baveystock CM, Parnell H et al. (1991) Randomised controlled trial of the effectiveness of a respiratory health worker in reducing impairment, disability and handicap due to chronic airflow limitation. *Thorax.* **46**: 559–64.

7   Littlejohns P, John AC. (1987) Auditory rehabilitation: should we listen to the patient? *British Medical Journal.* **294**: 1063–4.

8   Stewart-Brown S, Surender R, Bradlow J et al. (1995) The effects of fundholding in general practice on prescribing habits three years after introduction of the scheme. *British Medical Journal.* **311**: 1543–7.

9   Ham C. (1994) The future of purchasing: tolerance of diversity will be necessary. *British Medical Journal.* **309**: 1032–3.

2

What is a primary care-led health policy?

Andrew Harris

Most executive letters (ELs) containing guidance from the NHS Executive are destined to bureaucratic obscurity. Not so EL(94)79, Towards a primary care-led NHS. This has generated an enormous debate, a whole industry of conferences, and a myriad of speeches, articles and books. Unfortunately this has not led to a greater clarity. There remains a mixture of reactions from the enthusiastic, through the cynical to the defensive. This is partly due to weariness and low morale amongst the frontline staff caring for patients in a service experiencing an uncomfortable pace of change. In the main, however, it relates to confusion surrounding the policy itself. Indeed the very nature of health policy and its implementation need to be understood to judge the implications for GPs and other professionals and to see where it is leading.

Health care policy

Cynical commentators remark that the government has no policy, because the rationality and discreteness of its edicts cannot be discerned. If we accept Ignatieff's view[1] that policy is the selection of non-contradictory means to achieve non-contradictory ends over the medium to long-term, and Seedhouse's analysis[2] that a policy of purchasing services from a limited budget is simply not compatible with a policy of meeting needs regardless of ability to pay, we will inevitably conclude that the UK has no real health policy. However in a recent, timely and thought-provoking book,[3] policy is described as a series of more or less related activities and their intended and unintended consequences for those concerned. In the field of health planning there is a spectrum of approaches, with an academic debate between the extremes: rationalists[4] adopt a logical, standard, comprehensive approach, considering all the options to reach long-term goals; incrementalists,[5] take small steps, based on considering only a few close options, and ensure a few critical people are supportive. Doctors tend to feel comfortable with the rationalist approach, which is about how things ought to be; but it is often impractical, neglecting political and other stakeholder interactions, and is biased to the powerful vested interests of the medical profession. On the other hand incrementalism is more pluralistic and decentralized and focuses on how things are, but often obscures values and is less good at making the critical decisions for the future. Is the introduction of a primary care-led NHS a product of rationalism or incrementalism, or an intermediate process of both, so called 'mixed scanning'?[6]

Does it really matter?

It does, because it will tell us how best to respond to the policy. Kingdon[7] identified policy making as linear: agenda setting, identification of alternatives, authoritative choice and implementation of the decision. However the circumstances for policy implementation to perfectly achieve its objectives, never remotely apply in health services, and suggest that successful health policy making is anything but linear.

Thus Walt[8] suggests that frontline staff may change the way a policy is implemented, or even redefine the objectives, because they are closer to the problem and local situation. The greater the extent that the policy is rationalistic, with clearly stated objectives and vision, the easier it will be for support or for an offensive to be mounted, and the greater is the loss of political credibility if concessions are made to the implementors. The greater the extent that the policy is incrementally changing, with support in some quarters, and a lack of clear long-term vision, the greater the chance that some desired change will be made, without opposition, but the more likely that the precise nature and direction of that change will be determined by the implementors.

So what is this primary care-led policy which is both malleable and pioneering? Surprisingly little is said in the original executive letter, nor in the subsequent accountability framework. Firstly it is about *where decisions are made*: there is a stated intention for 'decisions about purchasing and providing health care to be taken as much as possible by GPs working closely with patients through primary health care teams'. It introduces the now familiar extensions of fundholding— community, standard and total purchasing (Table 2.1).

Table 2.1 New forms of fundholding.

	Community (3000+)	Standard (5000+)	Total
Purchasing	Staff, drugs, diagnostic tests, community health services	Community + virtually all elective surgery, outpatients	All hospital and community services, including A&E
Entry and operational requirements	Less than standard	Computers; management, public, financial and clinical accountability	52 pilots, acting in consortia, formal evaluation

It signals a new, strategic role for health authorities (which are now newly-constituted merged District and Family Health Service Authorities) 'to ensure that national and local priorities are met through GP led purchasing'.

Secondly it is about *strengthening relationships*: it plans development of strategic partnerships between health authorities and fundholding and non-fundholding GPs, and states 'all GPs, whether fundholding or not, will be more involved in developing local health strategies'.

What it will mean for non-fundholders is not described. One senior manager describes it as a 'fundamental shift away from publicly managed NHS hospitals to privately owned surgeries, from highly qualified consultants to local businessmen'.[3] This radical paradigm is likely to be one that unites many purchasing authority managers and hospital consultants who may be fearful of shifting power away from themselves. But this view of the policy reflects the intellectual leadership of Wessex Regional Health Authority, where two years of partnership between the profession and management led to the Wessex Framework for Primary Care. This, in turn, led to a significant shift of hospital services to community settings and established the capacity of primary care to be the principal focus of responsibility for health. This is the third aim of a primary care-led NHS; to focus on the *process of delivery of care*.

Why now?

So why is this poorly-defined, new policy being keenly promoted by the government? Is this a departure from previous policy trends, a dramatic shift in power and responsibility as Meads sees it, or a logical continuation or inevitable consequence of the NHS reforms thus far? Indeed, given the unpopularity of the government's policies on health, and the pace of imposed change, why introduce another reform? The answers are international and transcend party politics. They lie in the problems facing all developed countries seeking to achieve an affordably effective health service (Table 2.2).

All the factors in the table conspire to put enormous pressure on national governments, especially democratic developed countries, to increase health spending. Sixty years ago health care represented less than 1% of gross national product; now developed countries are spending between 6% and 11%. Service economies are becoming transnational, for example, 256 hospitals in Japan are managed and maintained by a Chicago based maintenance company.

Western economies are becoming knowledge intensive, rather than labour intensive, with implications for large organizations. They will have to reduce layers of management and focus on information needed to achieve clear strategic goals. The pace of technological change is phenomenal. For the advances in scientific knowledge to be applied successfully to population health, we need to find ways of both harnessing the explosion of commercial interest in biological sciences, as well as freeing up the public sector to promote entrepreneurial service developments. We also need to acknowledge that in affluent countries further major improvements in population health depend on lifestyle changes, better diet and housing, safer transport and greater employment. The contributions that health services,

Table 2.2 Factors driving countries for new paradigms of health care. (Adapted from Green A. (1992) *An introduction to health planning in developing countries.* Oxford University Press, Oxford.)

Factor	Impact on population
Demographic changes	Increased percentage of frail elderly; increased percentage productive employed
International economy	Recession increased government spending; affluence increased demand for health care
Medical technological advances	Scientific discovery, e.g. human genome project and new health products outstrip ability to pay
Information technology explosion	Increased demand for openness and sharing information; access to services via modern communication media
Consumer expectations	Increased complaints/litigation; increased demand for accountable services with explicit standards/outcomes
Power of medical professions	Generate new demand; resist change/disinvestment in unacceptable, inefficient or ineffective care
Changes in morbidity	Increased percentage of resources on chronic diseases, rather than acute cure
Health cost escalation	Health costs especially labour, exceed general retail price index

and hospital services in particular, can make to this, are limited. Against this background the medical profession clamours for more resources whilst research indicates that many medical interventions are not of proven effectiveness and drug costs continue to escalate. Small wonder that national governments are determined to find ways of controlling the increasing health care expenditure. The comparative success of the UK in containing health care costs masks the need to find stable and acceptable methods of control.

Countries with highly developed primary care services tend to have lower costs without affecting the levels of morbidity and mortality. In the British system, general practice is seen as the gatekeeper to the NHS, and thus a key to controlling demand in the rest of the system. So the case for primary care taking responsibility for cost containment decisions is very attractive to the policy maker and politician. With this in mind let us set the UK primary care-led policy in the context of the overall NHS reforms (Table 2.3).

The increasing influence of general management

This chronology shows the inexorable rise of management as a lever for change, for increasing professional accountability and delegating cost control. The primary care-led policy appears firstly to be the culmination of increasing interest in community and primary care as a key means of achieving the government's laudable public health objectives such as Health of the Nation. Secondly it is the inevitable

Table 2.3 The British health reforms affecting primary care.

Date	Reform	Objective	Impact
1966	The GP Charter (RCGP)	Safeguard clinical freedom and identity of GP as generalist	New models of care; wide variation in standards; GP dominates primary health care team; underinvestment in city practices
1974	Community health services transferred from local authority to NHS	Better co-ordination of primary and community health care	Improved standards; stronger links with hospital departments; practice attached staff
1974	Hospital boards abolished, family practitioner committees (FPCs) came under new area health authorities (AHA)	Reduce separation of primary and secondary care management; plan was US inspired bureaucracy	Unsuccessful, top heavy; FPCs were reactive, administering national contracts (GP etc.)
1974	Introduction of teams of managers and a new planning system	Speed up ability of NHS to react to changing needs of the population	Failure of consensus management in cash strapped service
1982	Abolish AHA, FPCs report to DHA; income generation schemes	Political expediency; cost containment	Some increased accountability of FPCs to DHA; few savings
1983	Griffiths enquiry: new central NHS Board and accountable general managers	Improve efficiency and value for money	Management key lever of change; clinician accountability to management
1985	HAs had to contract out laundry and catering	Competition to push down costs	Some savings
1986	Resource management and waiting list initiatives in hospitals	Improve information technology, decreased waiting, bypass bureaucrat by direct funding hospitals	Increased management skills of clinical leaders; 30% hospitals no resource management in 1995
1989	White Paper	Increased efficiency; increased patient choice; rewards for response to local need	Criticism and alarm about feasibility and appropriateness of untested market reforms
1990	New GP contract	Increased consumer and managerial accountability	Increased shift from GP to practice; increased prevention demotivation, and increased bureaucracy; attitude change to clinical freedom
1990	NHS and Community Care Act; internal market; purchaser–provider split, trusts, CHCs, community care	FHSAs/DHAs to balance needs of population and stakeholder views to drive change; HAs and LAs manage fixed budgets;: promote care in community rather than hospitals	Service turmoil, culture change, increased account-ability and increased efficiency; increased day surgery; inadequacy of information for contracting; management power

Table 2.3 Continued

Date	Reform	Objective	Impact
1990	GP fundholding	GP fundholders manage cash limited budgets as purchasers; reluctantly added late to reforms	Innovative care models; increased responsiveness of secondary sector; lower referrals; increased transaction costs; inequity
1992	Health of the Nation; first national health strategy	To focus on population health objectives	Increased health promotion; renaissance in public health; performance monitoring beyond process measures
1993	NHS R&D strategy and director (Peckham)	Focus on effectiveness and application of research in service	Struggles to use outcome measurement and disinvestments in ineffective care in service; evidence-based medicine and guidelines
1993	Patient's Charter	Focus on acceptability to consumer	Manipulation of waiting lists; some customer friendly organizations
1995	NHS Act: abolished RHAs, merged DHAs and FHSAs, some more NHS Executive control	To reduce bureaucracy and management costs; to integrate primary and secondary care; to give greater NHS Executive accountability	Decreased senior management with primary care experience; better joint DHA/FHSA working; increased involvement of GPs in commissioning

consequence of a politically dominated system in which management was viewed as slow to deliver and the medical profession as slow to change its practice. Doctors are the principal contributor to escalating health care expenditure; they are held in good esteem by the public, who value especially the personal care tradition of general practice. By making the primary care professional responsible for resource allocation in substantial parts of the secondary sector, the real rationing and priority choices will be made close to the patient by generalists. They bring professionally informed views of expensive hospital practice, and of the potential of primary care service pattern changes, and should be more acceptable to the public as resource allocators.

Who is in control?

Stories circulate that the policy was a finesse by the Department of Health civil service over the Management Executive, who had been recruited largely from outside their ranks, and had eclipsed the traditional power of the civil service. The argument goes that the Treasury were persuaded by the policy to devolve budget management to the NHS gatekeepers, and the civil servants gained new influence through their control of the General Medical Services Contract and so the Executive lost leverage through the handover of power from DHA managers to general practice. No doubt too the politicians were attracted by the philosophical justification of increasing the role of the private sector in the health care system. As Meads puts it 'on the back of primary care development the modern NHS has become a mixed economy'. But whatever the politics, the overriding concern of government is to delegate away from itself the difficult spending and saving decisions which contain costs: hence in giving money to doctors, not administrators. The primary care-led policy is a challenge and an opportunity to see whether those in white coats and uniforms can do better than those in grey suits in managing limited resources to the best benefit of the population.

The role of fundholding

In saying that the policy was an inevitable consequence of Treasury dominance does not mean that there are not other alternatives. The government could have gone for simply rolling out fundholding. However the initial ability to hold down prescribing costs better than non-fundholders has not been sustained. A prospective observational study of first wave fundholders has shown a failure to curb prescribing costs more effectively than non-fundholders in the long-term. Although much beneficial change has been claimed, the NHS Executive-commissioned Scottish evaluation of fundholding shadow project has only shown a major difference from non-fundholders in reduction of use of hospital consultant services. Fundholding's embarrassing underspends, high transaction costs, perennial inequitable funding process and the greater accessibility of services of fundholders, creating a two-tier service, have led to the political costs in the run up to the election being judged as too high.

What are the implications of this policy for primary care shift?

There are eight key areas.

Responsibility for prioritizing spending

GPs will have to face the reality of deciding whether or not to take some responsibility for rationing and priority setting for their patients. It is widely held that a perceived conflict of interest for GPs taking on this role is the prime reason for opposition to fundholding. There is little doubt that budget holding brings power to effect change, but also brings the responsibility for deciding priorities. Those GPs who elect to ensure that the rationing decisions are another's responsibility, should be entitled to a major influence on that process, but will have to accept that the comfort of not sharing that responsibility will leave them with less power. Nevertheless significant achievements have been made in service change by GP-sensitized DHA purchasing. Who are the appropriate people and what skills and experience do they need to set priorities? What level is appropriate for this process; should it be in primary care itself, at the lowest possible level? Whose views should be taken into account and how? And what values and principles should underlie such decisions?

Some decisions have to be taken at a large population level, such as establishing specialist treatment or residential units or mounting screening programmes; but many decisions on service development cannot be taken at a macro level, partly because of the remoteness from the patient and partly because the clinical and academic skills are not there. Much is to commend doctors gaining management skills, but it is personal skills, attitude and understanding of complex issues, rather than background discipline, which matter most. There is not scope here to discuss the underlying values and philosophical basis of resource allocation decisions, save to say that they seldom are, but should be made, explicit. A local democratic legitimacy should be gained for their adoption, and decision makers should be held accountable for their application. Suggested principles are laid out in Boxes 2.1 and 2.2.

Box 2.1   Suggested principles for primary and community care.

- Appropriateness (which site, which professional and which standard)

- Value for money

- Patient empowering (health education, reducing demand and utilization of services)

- Social acceptability

- Accessibility

- Maximization of evidence-based practice

Box 2.2   Suggested principles for secondary care (adapted from Maxwell)[9]

- Maximization of effectiveness and monitoring of outcomes

- Equity (geographic, client and type of purchaser)

- Social acceptability (including fully informed consent)

- Efficiency (cost, communication, risk management)

- Responsiveness to primary care

- Reflects epidemiologically-based need

Substitution and controlling the shift from secondary sector to primary care

There is the opportunity to control the pace of substitution or shift across the secondary primary sector interface, and to define primary and community care in its own right, and not just as a residue of what the hospitals cannot or will not shed. For too long, general practice and community health services have been at the receiving end of changes outside their control: the closure of long-stay institutions, the failures of community care, the inappropriately early hospital discharge, and delegation of specialist drug monitoring, have generated extra work without adequate training and resources to match these new challenges. By controlling purchasing from primary care both professional and financial power will be together and create a more balanced partnership with the powerful vested interests of the hospital specialists. Given the historic underfunding of capital investment in primary care (for example, in Birmingham £500m was committed to hospital development and £5m to FHSAs for primary care development) this may involve saying 'no' to service transfers without accompanying funding, or radically changing service provision.

Responsiveness to population need and accountability

For whom is primary care purchasing or leading the service? This may seem an obvious question to a GP, who will probably answer 'my registered patients', and to a community health trust, which will probably say 'the population in our geographic area'. The disjunctions in commissioning of primary and community care have been highlighted and urgently need addressing. The sum of general practice lists is very different from the local population, defined by the census, and both probably vary significantly, in inner city areas and where there is high mobility, from reality (Table 2.4).

Table 2.4   How populations vary from real population (+ or –) according to denominator used.

Example	GP list	Census
Homeless	–	–
Absent student	+	+
Recent move		–
Not on census as fear of poll tax		–
Never properly GP registered	–	+
Recently left GP but not area	+	
Temporary resident	+	

These differences are not merely academic, as the population determines the information on which purchasing decisions are made, defines the nature of responsiveness and determines accountability. Robson[10] has elegantly shown the need to define core practice populations to enable comparative audit. Health authorities have difficulties in defining locality purchasing and stress the need for clarity of objectives and sharing intelligence. Furthermore, who represents the patient when the GP is the provider and how will GPs' fitness to purchase care be assessed?

GP fundholders are required to be accountable to management, patients and the wider public, both financially and professionally. This entails involving patients in service planning, publishing information and having performance monitored. Is this the sort of model a new non-fundholding primary care-led service would use? From a public health point of view responsiveness to the health strategy of the district health authority and to the local authority strategic plans, and a recognition of need in the population rather than just those who are currently using the service is essential. This requires a cultural shift of significant proportion in a workforce overwhelmed by patient demand, in which being asked to consider needs of the non-consulting population seems a futile exercise.

Yet are we happy that a chronically neurotic woman with a marital problem occupies as much of her GP's time as it would take him/her to do domiciliary visits and perform annual diabetic checks on non-attenders? Is it ethical that mothers with no risk factors receive frequent antenatal checks (of doubtful effectiveness) whilst a Vietnamese community with a high risk of hepatitis has not had screening or protection? Should nurses be screening opportunistically all attenders for diabetes (on equivocal evidence) whilst the majority of the elderly population suffer disability from hearing loss without adequate hearing assessment or provision of aids and education? If primary care is expected to give an important contribution to achieving Health of the Nation targets or local health strategy, how can it do so, whilst dominated by a reactive style of practice? These are questions about relative need. The feasibility and place of primary care needs assessment has been extensively reviewed but it seems that very few fundholder or non-fundholder commissioning decisions have been informed by a needs assessment or public health input.[11] There is a need to select key areas where needs-driven decisions are crucial to prevent minority and 'Cinderella needs' being overshadowed by powerful patient and professional demands in other areas. It seems likely that much available quantitative information will apply to groups or populations different from those for which responsibility for purchasing is held, and that the wealth of practice held information has qualitative value, but that both are difficult to relate to decisions about resource allocation. Making sense of this will require close co-operation between primary care and public health and some convergence of roles.

General practice's ability to deliver

The above questions are also questions about capability. Developing a model to enable the primary health care team to respond to local needs efficiently and effectively, requires commitment of resources, development of leaders, teambuilding and training in management and public health tasks. We cannot divorce the development of primary care as providers from the process of its purchasing secondary care.

Historically, improving general practice has operated through feedback loops from incentives for individual general practitioners, which is now inappropriate for primary health care team development. General practice partnerships are mostly 'people orientated', in which individuals are the central point; the power base is the medical expertise and organizational goals are usually subordinate, requiring mutual consent. Such cultures are severely tested as the size and complexity of practices grow. The degree of adaptability and teamwork required in modern general practice, and especially for primary care-led purchasing, will require evolution, perhaps particularly into task cultures. In these organizations there is not the hierarchy of the traditional bureaucratic role cultures, but a matrix organization in which influence is widely spread and high degrees of control are exercised by all workers; and the roles are flexible, bringing in the right people with the right skills at the right time.

Central versus local contracts

This change will require both attitudinal change as well as reform of the antiquated, nationally negotiated general medical services contracting system. Amendments and add-ons developed by local FHSAs and in the London Implementation Zone have begun incrementally to introduce some flexibility. Despite formal BMA opposition, the likelihood of diverse local contracts with practices emerging seems high. General practice should welcome this, since the relationship with the new health agencies could become a more distant one of setting broad objectives and monitoring. In exchange for accepting that degree of accountability, practices could have greater freedom to shape their own services and those they buy, sensitive to local demand and need. This approach seems to fit with the attraction even to non-fundholders of the fundholder freedom to vire across budgets. It is interesting to note the professional stances taken in the primary care development simulation exercise carried out in Bath.[3] The professional organizations such as the GMSC were keen to change national and local rules to allow for broader primary health care teams and multidisciplinary partnership organizations, with freedom to contract with other practitioners and to generate some income by charging. The non-fundholding GPs were keen to establish locality models, incorporating health and social care, but felt there were enormous obstacles for achieving change, principally lack of time to think and a hugely conservative workforce. So perhaps one of the messages of the opportunity presented by primary care purchasing might be for GPs to take protected time away from patients, to develop a vision and dare to believe it is possible.

Re-examination of roles in the primary care team

The fifth implication of a successful primary care-led service arises out of the capability and vision discussed above. It is no less radical or liberating, and is the re-examination of the role of the doctor, and in particular the general practitioner. The medical profession in the UK established self control of training requirements, entry and self regulation through the Medical Act of 1858, well before the establishment of the welfare state or the rise of management. They defined the validity of medical scientific knowledge, resisted its codification and public dissemination, creating an indetermination of knowledge that disempowered the consumer. In primary care this generated a role of individual advocacy on behalf of patients. Yet this very concentration of power has had the disadvantage of embracing within general medical practice role overload and role conflict. An example is the tension between that of advocacy on behalf of the individual patient and the executive decisions to prioritize services or ration resources. The Royal College of General Practitioners has highlighted the need for GPs to resolve the tensions in their biomedical, biographical, anticipatory and consumerist roles. King's Fund workshops with general practitioners demonstrated there are contemporarily four elements to the GP role.[12] These indicate the benefits of reducing tensions by specialization and role differentiation within practices (Table 2.5).

Table 2.5 Potential role differentiation in general medical practice.

Clinical servant	Clinical care, education and research
Health counsellor	Personal decision consultant and patient advocate; lobbyist and network manager
Chief executive officer	Corporate expression of general practice; negotiate contracts and service agreements
Care shaper/development manager	Change agent across boundaries; meeting client group needs; translates strategy; develops clinical services in organizations

A model which has put into practice the best use of individual skills in their primary health care team is the Lyme Regis project, where public service values and private sector initiatives were linked with the needs of different stakeholders. Certainly modest initiatives can be taken in all practices in looking at the relative roles of doctor, practice manager and nurse, and in most, there is greater scope for delegation, realignment and clarification of what each can best do. Many of the traditional GP clinical services such as provision and explanation of treatments may be better shared with nursing staff. Extended role nurses with their own list is an example of such developments being piloted. Many members of the primary care team, such as the manager, health visitor or pharmacist may have skills that are not being fully exploited. Put simply, GPs cannot control or do all the key tasks of a modern primary care practice, and individuals should be focused on what would most fulfil them.

Within the secondary sector an equally fundamental rethink of professional and managerial roles is required. In a primary care-led NHS, the consultant in many specialties may need to evolve into an educator, coach, assessor; focusing on standards and supporting primary care to do most of the actual provision of service. Fundholders are now contracting for direct telephone advice; video telephone diagnosis is being piloted; ambulatory paediatric care is being set up; outreach clinics are being evaluated.

Resources have not flowed adequately into primary care to support substitution of services from hospitals. Part of the reason is that the NHS accounting and information systems are still focused on secondary care; on finished consultant episodes and bed days. The challenge for primary care-led commissioning is to both change professional attitudes within hospitals and the contracting currency. These developments have to be designed in an environment in which increasing information and empowerment is being made available to users of the service.

Diversity and how to address poor quality

To those for whom this sounds a distant radical agenda, unlike their own practice – grow your own vision. One of the strengths of British general practice is its diversity. The nature of practice in the Dales will rightly be very different from the East End of London. This diversity however cannot be allowed to be a cloak for unacceptable variations in quality of practice, which continue to need addressing by a combination of organizational development, investment, audit, performance monitoring and professional assessment and retraining. Our health service man-power is a scarce and demoralized resource. We should build upon the skills and motivations of those in the service, supplementing them where necessary, devel-oping new roles; and not be fearful if one GP has a very different looking job from another, or one practice or primary care unit is financed or managed differently. There must be a health authority-led primary and community care strategy which has some clear principles and goals about accessibility, equity, responsiveness etc. This should encourage imaginative and innovative partnerships with the private sector, voluntary sector or community trusts. The latter could be contracted as a major facilities support for staff and resource management for general practice, and general practice could be contracted to provide specified additional services by the trusts.

Development agencies

Partnerships could form between academic departments, consultancies and trusts to form development agencies, which could be given the bulk of the health agency primary care development budget, together with the staff whose expertise is in provider development. This would slim down the health authority and put the change agents closer to the field, and in a better position to influence opinion leaders, without conflict of interest. These new agencies could then support and develop practices (particularly small areas) within a strategic context set by the commissioning agency. Alternatively groups of practices could form locality units to lead development and perhaps purchase from community trusts. As the new world unfolds, hopefully GPs will not feel that they are losing control by ceding the employment of staff to organizations better able to flexibly manage and recruit staff, if the gains are wider influence over the whole primary care development agenda, and an extension of services accessible to their patients without attending hospital. The options to develop one-stop shops with social services and specialist community trust staff, outpatient, polyclinic and resource centres for primary health care teams, or new models of out-of-hours care are exciting. These require imagination beyond the typical patterns of provision and a spirit of trust and partnership rather than competition between primary care providers.

Managing demand

None of this is possible if primary care cannot control its workload better; that is manage demand. This is the seventh and perhaps most critical of the implications of primary care-led service. Current stresses in frontline staff are so high, that unless the capacity issue in primary and community health care is urgently addressed, there will be no capability to develop or purchase imaginatively or responsively. The reasons for the increased demand are many and varied; some are shown in Table 2.6.

Table 2.6 Some causes of increased demand for primary and community health care.

Underlying cause	Impact
Government policy, e.g. charters, media	Raised consumer expectations
Social trends in employment and leisure	Higher patient mobility
Cash limited local authority community care	Increasing role in managing complex problems in mentally ill, disabled
Pressure on secondary sector budgets	Earlier hospital discharge
Demographic trends	More frail elderly
Successful international research	Drug and treatment advances
Consumer, nurse and government enthusiasm	Hospital-at-home role
Unemployment, changing role of women and family structure	High consultation rates
Reduction in hospital beds	Greater difficulty in arranging admissions
Contracting system increases administration burden	Less doctor time with patients

Trying to lead purchasing or service development for the NHS from primary care without efficient management of demand, is not only foolhardy, but irresponsible, because it puts much of the responsibility for service inadequacies on patients, without equipping them to make appropriate judgements in the light of their need, that of others, and available resources. Some suggestions for management are shown in Box 2.3.

The workload of UK ambulatory care is 3.3 annual person consultation rate compared with 3.0 for US family physicians, but interestingly the weekly volume of direct patient–physician contacts in the US is higher and more widely distributed than in the UK, where average consultation times are three and a half minutes shorter.[13] This suggests there may be opportunities for looking critically at increasing the doctor–patient time, by freeing British doctors of other tasks, and using it to improve the self-coping mechanisms of patients. However it should not be

---

Box 2.3 Suggestions for demand management.

- Patient education initiatives on service utilization and use of non-statutory supports

- Non-doctors taking over parts of medical role, especially nurses, psychologists, pharmacists

- Training GPs and practice managers in efficient performance in organizations

- Training GPs in risk management

- Training in teamwork development

- New out-of-hours initiatives: co-ops, centres, telephone advice, 24 hour nurse/psychology/pharmacy/social work

- Audits and comparison of consultations and referrals with peers

- Appropriate and timely patient information, acceptable to minority groups, new patients

- Establishment of patient groups

- Use of volunteers and lay workers

- Support, respite and training for carers

- Control through monitoring, joint policies and contracts, substitution of work from the hospital

- Minimize but improve validity of information and data collected and distributed; policy on usage/access

---

forgotten that the UK system is both more equitable and cheaper: half as cheap per GDP% and per capita costs, for similar outcomes and processes.

Education and training

In conclusion there are a number of areas on which practices need to focus, asking themselves, what are we doing now, what do we want to do, and how do we get there? They are insufficient without the recognition that none of this is possible without initial education of those involved and an ongoing training and development programme. The eight key areas for primary care are summarized in Box 2.4.

Box 2.4 Summary of priorities for general practice in a primary care-led service.

- Agreement on responsibility for prioritizing service expenditure

- Controlling substitution and shift of work from secondary to primary care

- Responsiveness to population need and accountability to patients, the profession and managers

- Ability to deliver

- Re-examination of roles in the primary care team

- Diversity and how to address poor quality

- Managing demand

- Education and training in primary care-led NHS; skilling, teambuilding, monitoring and developing

---

How will we know if it has been a success?

Carruthers has produced a list of criteria for success of total fundholding schemes.[14] Suggested criteria developed from this list, of importance to the broader primary care-led NHS, are shown in Table 2.7. Effective integration of primary, community and secondary services will require new methods of purchasing and handling the problems of disinvesting in institutional care.

Table 2.7 Evaluation of a primary care-led NHS.

Objective	Criteria
Effective integration of commissioning (embraces influencing, purchasing and contracting across sectors)	• Shared corporate objectives and purchasing intentions • Targets in strategy for disinvestment from hospital care • Measures of health and critical social need, e.g. damp housing
Better partnerships with other organizations	• General practice/community trust/LA social service departments, shared care management approach • Responsiveness to each others' priorities • Joint in-service training
Explicit responsibility for decision making	• Clarity of organizational aims and objectives

Table 2.7   Continued

Objective	Criteria
	• Explicitness about responsibility for prioritization of resource allocation, and rationing decisions
	• Process of gaining local consent to values and principles underlying decisions
Value for money	• Transaction costs of different providers and systems
	• Specific measures of costs and benefit of shift of service from secondary to primary care
Responses to population need	• In stable populations use of needs assessment and patient outcomes
	• Contribution to Health of the Nation and national objectives
Accountability to management and patient	• Action plans for poor quality providers or services
	• Doctor–patient contact time
	• Openness with users about comparative outcomes
	• Adequate quality of information
Efficient provisioh of appropriate care	• Reduction in duplication, e.g. GP/CHS clinics
	• Use of appropriate professional, according to local protocols and reprofiling
Maximization of evidence-based interventions	• Monitoring use of known effective interventions and reasons for variations
	• Explicit multi-disciplinary clinical audit results linked to changes in service and referral
Management of demand	• Monitoring trends in service utilization, pre and post, and across areas
Equity of health care delivery	• Equitable resource allocation to providers

Table 2.7   Continued

Objective	Criteria
	• Monitor users over time
	• Needs assessment in key areas
Sustainability and stability of need systems	• Development of new 'champions' and opinion leaders
	• Proactivity and capability to respond to changes externally
	• Broad ownership by primary health care team
Staff retention and recruitment	• Filled vacancies
	• Retention of local trainees

The experience of Castlefields health centre in developing the care manager function is instructive; creating opportunities to evaluate interagency co-ordination and trends in social and health needs.

Harris identified five characteristics for judging strategic competence:[15]

1   principles

2   timescale/pace

3   comprehensiveness

4   coherence

5   revision.

Additional measures of the implementation process and impacts of service change are needed. Critical to the validity of evaluations will be baseline antecedent measures specific to the time and place of the service management changes, and proper consideration of conflicting objectives of different stakeholders.

Better partnerships with other organizations are crucial, particularly community trusts and local authority social service departments, and the key hospital departments of psychiatry and geriatrics. It is of interest that in reviewing teamwork in mental health, it was found that the two keys to success were secondary care providers' responsiveness to individual primary care views, and GP willingness to temper their preferences based on personal experience with research evidence on the options. The interrelation between health authorities, provider units and primary care teams is such that any evaluation process has to apply to all three. A key issue will be value for money and it is crucial to compare transaction costs of fundholder, DHA and new emerging models of purchasing. For total practice fundholders with stable populations such as the Worth Valley, the opportunities to measure need and patient outcomes is a real one, but such pilots are already finding the restriction of current information systems.

The importance of ensuring costs incurred in transfer of services from secondary sector are less than savings made, leads to three key measures of evaluation of such shifts:

1   replacement of hospital activity lost

2   hospital resource management to a reduced total cost base

3   individual general practice resource consequences of clinical guidelines.

Finally a Consumer Association survey suggests the provider role of fundholding general practices has deteriorated in quality; a reminder that monitoring patient outcomes and perceptions of trends is crucial. Time spent with patients is probably a simple and telling measure. Starfield[16] has devised a score to compare international primary care systems. This shows the UK in a strong position (score 1.7) compared with the US (0.2). There is general concordance between the primary care score, health indicators and peoples' satisfaction; which are all high in the Netherlands (1.5).

The UK, despite a high score, has a low ranking for health indices and an intermediate one for satisfaction, perhaps due to underfunding hospital care, education or social service. Starfield also found that use of technology and number of subspecialties best predicted high expenditure. In comparing different service models these variables, as well as the trend in Starfield's score, can be used in evaluation. But political courage will be needed to foster proper evaluations in the context of differential funding.

Conclusions

This colossal agenda is a real opportunity for primary care that may never happen again. Much of what has been discussed is about defining the central principle of primary and community care, namely appropriateness. This is about using knowledge of effectiveness of interventions, efficiency, patient acceptability and clinical experience, to establish appropriate normative practice. Its main components are who is the most appropriate person to provide each service and at what location and to what standard should it be provided? It can be seen that public health skills, managerial experience and user input are all crucial to this experience. But for the first time primary care has centre stage to shape the service. It must be clear where responsibility, particularly budgetary, begins and ends. It needs to have a clear set of objectives, a robust commissioned evaluation and a proper sense of mutual respect for all professionals working in primary and community care. The workforce of the NHS are its most precious asset, but the jewels in the crown need to be very bright for all to see their value.

References

1 Ignatieff M. (1992) The grey emptiness inside John Major. *The Observer,* 15 November: 25.

2 Seedhouse D. (1994) Real government required. *Health Care Analysis.* **2**: 1–4.

3 Robinson R, Huntingdon J, Meads G (eds). (1995) *The Primary Care Challenge.* Churchill Livingstone, Edinburgh.

4 Berry DE. (1974) The transfer of planning theories to health planning practice. *Policy Sciences.* **5**.

5 Lindblom (1959) The science of muddling through. *Public Administration Review.* **19**: 79–88.

6 Etzioni A. (1967) Mixed Scanning: a third approach to decision making. *Public Administration Review.* **27**: 385–92.

7 Kingdon J. (1984) *Agendas, alternatives and public policies.* Little Brown & Co., Boston.

8 Walt G. (1994) *Health Policy: an introduction to process and power.* Witwatersrand University Press, Johannesburg.

9 Maxwell RJ. (1992) Dimensions of quality revisited: from thought to action. *Quality in Health Care.* 171–7.

10 Robson J, Falshaw M and the Healthy Eastender Project. (1995) Audit of preventive activities in 16 inner London practices using a validated measure of patient population, the active patient denominator. *British Journal of General Practice.* **45**: 403–6.

11 Harris A. (1996) *Needs to Know: a guide to primary care needs assessment.* Churchill Livingstone, Edinburgh. In press.

12 Harris A. (1995) Fresh fields: the relationship between public health medicine and general medical practice. *Primary Care Management.* **5**: 7.

13 Fry J, Light D and Rodnick J. (1995) *Reviving Primary Care: a US–UK comparison.* 118–40. Radcliffe Medical Press, Oxford.

14 Carruthers I. (1994) Total fundholding in the mainstream of the NHS. *Primary Care Management.* **4**: 7–9.

15 Harris A. (1994) How should changes in primary health care be evaluated? In *Controversies in Health Care Policies: challenges to practice* (ed. M Marinker), BMJ Publishing Group, London.

16 Starfield B. (1992) *Primary Care: concept, evaluation and policy.* Oxford University Press, New York.

3

Information for a primary care-led health service – health needs assessment

John Shanks and Tim Crayford

> *Health needs assessment is just a more systematic way of trying to answer the question: what sort of health services will be most useful?*

Principles

What are 'health needs'?

The term usually means 'need for health *service*'. The Department of Health defines need for health service as 'the ability to benefit' from that service. This is a deceptively simple definition which presumes that there is agreement on what benefit will be conferred by an intervention. This approach requires consideration of a range of different types of information. It makes a distinction from the demand for health services, as shown by the pattern of people who currently make use of services. There are four main aspects of the need for health services:

1   *demography and epidemiology.* What sort of people are in the population and what sort of health problems do they have?

2   *effectiveness.* How effective are the various possible treatments and services available?

3   *comparisons.* What differences or similarities are there from comparable populations elsewhere?

4   *the corporate view.* What are the preferences and priorities of local people?

An assessment of need attempts to go beyond current patterns of service usage to identify people who would be able to benefit from a service if they used it. For a practice, this could imply taking account of those people who are not registered with the practice but could be, those registered patients who do not use present services and those services which the practice could provide but currently does not. This might mean trying to assess the requirements of sub-groups of the population who are less likely to be registered with a GP (homeless people, refugees, drug misusers, people with severe mental illness) and also those patients whom the practice rarely sees.

Why develop a primary care-based method of health needs assessment?

A foundation for primary care-led purchasing
The current intention of the Department of Health is to move towards a primary care-led NHS. In particular, commissioning (or purchasing) of health services should be primary care-led. Earlier policy statements emphasized that commissioning decisions should be based as far as possible on some systematic assessment of the health needs of the population. In order to be consistent with primary care-led purchasing in a primary care-led NHS, the assessment of health needs should also be firmly based in primary care.

To reflect the great variability of small populations
Primary care services typically serve small populations of perhaps 5000–10 000 compared to the population of 200 000 or more which may be served by an acute general hospital. These small populations are much more variable than larger population units. Among the general practices of South East London, for example, the proportion of elderly people on the practice list varies from almost nil to 33%. This huge variation is much greater than any comparable differences between the areas covered by health commissioning authorities or health regions. If we are to develop health services which appropriately serve the varying needs of these small populations, then we must have an accurate picture of how needs differ between one practice and another, between one locality and another.

To make use of the richly detailed knowledge of primary care practitioners
Because primary care practitioners often maintain long-term contact with their patients, they have the opportunity to acquire detailed knowledge of patients' circumstances and preferences. Primary care practitioners may therefore be better able to represent the opinions of patients and also in a better position to obtain more detailed views from their patients to supplement the information passed on in the course of routine consultations.

Total or relative need?

It is probably impractical to attempt to assess all the needs for health services of any population. It is rarely possible to get enough information to make such a complete assessment and it is unlikely that there would ever be the resources to satisfy all needs. It may be more realistic to attempt to get a picture of relative need; perhaps by comparing one practice to another in an FHSA area or one local area to another. This relative ranking of need is often quite adequate for the purpose of setting priorities for allocation of limited resources for practice staffing, for example.

Sometimes a practice may be interested in getting an accurate picture of the need for one particular type of health service, for example, sexual health and contraceptive services for young people from an ethnic minority community. On other occasions, a new practice may wish to make a more general scan across a range of possible health needs to form a broader picture of the range of services which might be offered.

Needs met and unmet

Some of the needs identified by a needs assessment exercise will already have services in place to meet them. Others may be new needs, perhaps not recognized before or neglected in terms of service provision. By comparing the pattern of needs identified to the pattern of services currently provided it is possible to get a picture of gaps and overlaps – needs for which there appears to be no service (e.g. general medical services for single, homeless men) or needs for which several services seem to be fulfilling the same purpose (e.g. bereavement counselling from practice-based counsellors, palliative care teams, voluntary agencies and community mental health teams).

Practical examples

The ideal situation for assessing the needs of a practice population would be to have readily available a complete and standardized set of individual data on each person which would include key facts such as age, sex, social circumstances, health problems, current treatments, personal opinions and preferences. This is unattainable and likely to remain so. No current sources of information even come close to meeting these requirements. The following methods described are attempts to make use of what knowledge is currently available or readily obtainable. In order to do justice to the complexity of primary care services, a comprehensive strategy for needs assessment should include both quantitative and qualitative approaches.

Quantitative methods

These are approaches which rely on numerical data.

Geographical distribution of registered patients

Every patient on the practice list should have a postcode which allows their location to be mapped. Just looking at a map like this can immediately give an impression of the extent to which the practice population is compact and concentrated around the practice or widely scattered over a large area (Figure 3.1a, b). These two extremes imply quite different demands on the practice in terms of the likelihood of patients being able or willing to attend the surgery and the time taken up in home visiting. Many practices feel it is good for both patients and the practice to review the distribution of their list from time to time and perhaps to suggest that outlying patients who have moved further away should register with a nearer practice.

Age–sex distribution

The age–sex register is one of the simplest and most basic pieces of information, available to every practice, and yet it can yield a great deal of valuable information because the likelihood of a particular health problem is often largely determined by age or gender. Practices vary greatly in the mix of men and women, young and elderly, which they serve. This is only partly a reflection of the catchment area from which the practice draws patients; it also reflects how the practice is perceived by the community. So, a single-handed male practitioner will often have a list which is relatively deficient in young women and children (Figure 3.2a, b) perhaps because some women prefer to have the option of seeing a female practitioner or the facilities of a larger practice offering women's health and maternity services. Conversely, a practice which shares the same premises as community child health services may find that it attracts more than its share of young families (Figure 3.3a, b). In order to be able to derive maximum information for the age–sex register, it is necessary to make comparisons both with the average for the whole FHSA area and with the catchment area from which the practice draws patients. This last comparison requires information which goes beyond the list of patients actually registered, e.g. national census information.

Census data and deprivation

Every practice has available a simple measure of the extent of socioeconomic deprivation among its registered patients in terms of the numbers of patients (if any) who attract additional deprivation payments. These payments are nationally calculated on the basis of the Jarman score of the area in which each of the registered patients lives. The Jarman score was devised to estimate the extra workload which a practice could expect from dealing with certain types of patient (e.g. elderly, under-fives, people living alone etc.). These same factors which affect a practice's workload also reflect the social and economic factors which influence the health of the local population and so the Jarman score can be quite a convenient proxy measure for health. In general, the higher the Jarman score, the more deprived is the population and the poorer will be the state of general health. It is possible to analyse other information from the national census to build up a picture of the

a
Displayed population, 11 722

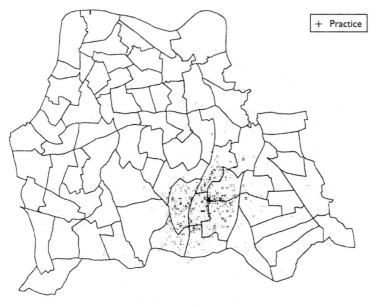

b
Displayed population 2234

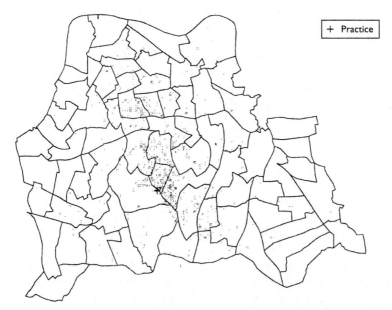

Figure 3.1a and b The geographic distribution of registered patients for two inner city practices. The boundaries are electoral wards. The practice in **a** has a relatively large list size with a very compact distribution around it while the practice in **b** has a much smaller list size which is thinly scattered over a much larger area.

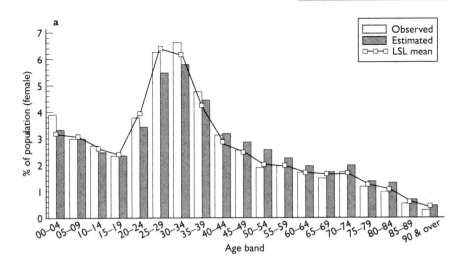

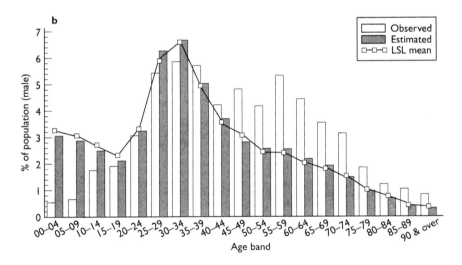

Figure 3.2a and b The age–sex distribution for the registered list of a single-handed male practitioner who has practised from the same premises for many years. Note the relative deficit of young women and children and the preponderence of elderly people on the list. 'Observed' is the actual mix of registered patients; 'estimated' is what would be expected from the composition of the population in the practice's catchment area; and 'LSL mean' is the average for the whole FHSA area.

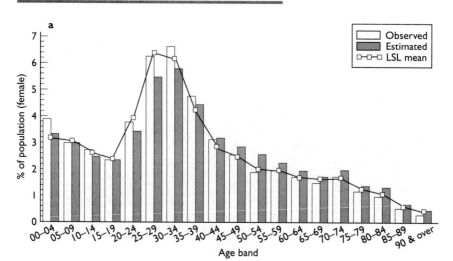

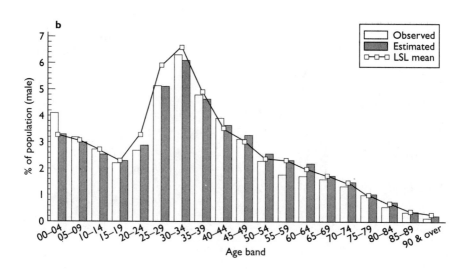

Figures 3.3a and b   The age–sex distribution for the registered list of a group practice with several female partners. Young women and young children are well represented on the list. 'Observed' is the actual mix of registered patients; 'estimated' is what would be expected from the composition of the population in the practice's catchment area; and 'LSL mean' is the average for the whole FHSA area.

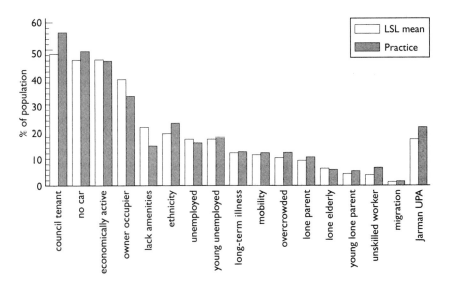

Figure 3.4 Attributed social characteristics of a practice population. This gives an estimate of the social characteristics which the list of registered patients would be expected to have if they are typical of the catchment area from which the practice draws its patients. For each characteristic, the predicted value for the practice population is compared to the average value for the FHSA area as a whole ('LSL mean'). These predicted values are derived from the answers which local people gave to the most recent national census in 1991. The practice shown here has a higher than average Jarman score which means it is serving a more than usually deprived population. The prediction is for higher than average proportions of people who are from ethnic minority groups, lone parents, council tenants, without access to a car or living in overcrowded accommodation.

expected social characteristics of a practice population (Figure 3.4). Because social factors have such a powerful influence on health this may help a practice to predict the sort of health problems it is particularly likely to see and what sort of services may be more useful in responding to these.

Prescribing data

Every practice now receives PACT data from the Prescription Pricing Authority and many practices can also generate additional prescribing information from their own computers. Information on prescribing has a dual function:

1   it provides a picture of one rather important type of clinical activity

2   it can in some cases act as a proxy marker for a particular health problem (e.g. one way to estimate the number of insulin-dependent diabetics would be to look at the number of people receiving a prescription for insulin).

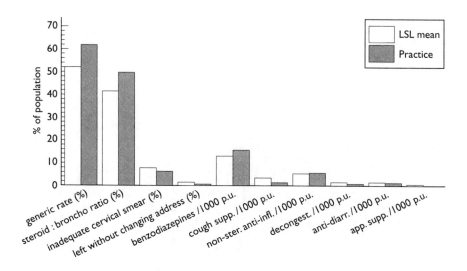

Figure 3.5   Set of indicators readily obtained from routine data on prescribing, patient registration and cervical screening. These help to highlight areas of practice activity which are going particularly well or which merit review. The value for the practice is compared in each case to the average value for the FHSA area as a whole ('LSL mean'). The first two indicators are conventional markers of good prescribing. In simple terms, the higher these values are the better. The other eight indicators are ones where lower values are usually better: the proportion of cervical smears which are returned as inadequate, the proportion of patients who leave the practice without changing address, the prescribing rate for a selection of drugs of 'limited therapeutic value' such as benzodiazepines, cough and appetite suppressants, systemic decongestants, anti-diarrhoeals and topical non-steroidal anti-inflammatory agents. For the practice examined here, most of the values are better than the local average with the exception of benzodiazepine prescribing which seems rather high. The practice used this information to review its benzodiazepine prescribing policy.

Attempts have been made to find convenient prescribing indicators which point to good or poor clinical practice (Figure 3.5). For example, the ratio of inhaled steroids to bronchodilators prescribed throws some light on how well the practice is managing asthmatics. This use of data is dealt with in more detail in chapter four.

Making use of data from the practice computer
Practice computer systems
Increasingly, practice-based computers are being used to store details of patients' medical histories. Compared to the sort of information which is centrally held by the FHSA, information from practice computers has the advantage of being up-to-date and capable of being related to individual patients. On the other hand, not every practice at present has the interest or capability to collect such information and those who do may use any one of a number of different systems of coding or storing the data.

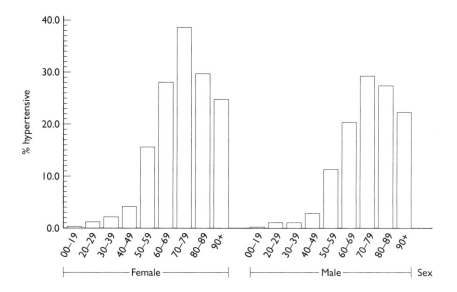

Figure 3.6   Age–sex specific rates for prescription with anti-hypertensive drugs.

Information from the practice computer can be used in a number of different ways:

- *monitor health of the practice population* (examine the frequency of health problems or risk factors)

- *audit* (describe and evaluate the use of treatments)

- *explore relationships between health and population factors* (examine whether particular subgroups of the practice population have particular health problems).

Figure 3.6 shows the age–sex specific rates of diagnosed and treated hypertension in one practice in south-east London. Note that in this practice, as in most others, men of all ages are less likely than women to be treated for hypertension. Clearly there are particular opportunities for measuring women's blood pressure in the course of family planning or ante-natal care. The extent of the male–female discrepancy in treated hypertension may help a practice decide whether it wishes to give more priority to finding ways of persuading men to have their blood pressure measured. Only information from the practice's own computer could allow this sort of analysis: PACT data cannot be related to individual patients and does not contain information about gender.

Figure 3.7 shows the age distribution of patients at one practice who had received one or more repeat prescriptions for benzodiazepines over a period of at least six weeks. The pattern suggests that there may be two distinct groups of patients: a young to middle-aged group (who turned out to be mainly on

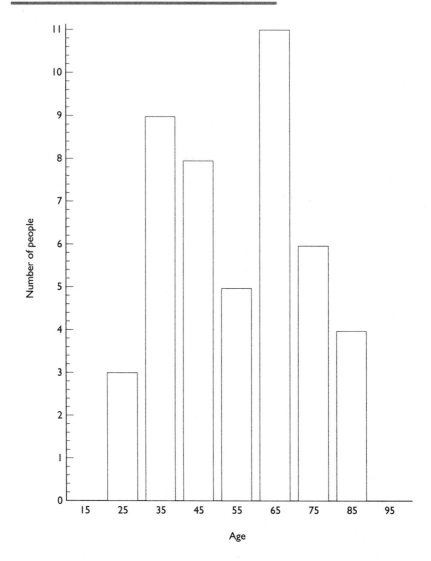

Figure 3.7 Age distribution of people who are taking benzodiazepines chronically.

anxiolytics) and an older group (who were identified as being mainly on hypnotics). The practice was able to make better plans to tackle long-term benzodiazepine use with this information.

How good is the information on practice computers?
The quality of the information stored on practice computers is very variable. Some GPs in a practice may be less methodical than others about entering diagnostic data. Information about contacts with other professionals in the practice team may not get entered at all. Locums may not understand the system. Details of home

visits may get missed out altogether. But some items of information do get reliably and completely entered. Most practices which use a computer at all make use of the facility to produce computer-generated prescriptions. Prescribing information therefore tends to be of quite good quality. The best incentive towards improving the quality of other information is for the practice to find it useful in its day-to-day activities. It is always easier to persuade people to take the trouble to collect information which they can see to be useful to them.

Effectiveness

Evidence-based practice

The definition of 'need' for a service as 'the ability to benefit' from that service implies that the effectiveness of the service must be an important consideration. There could be no need for a service which is ineffective because it would produce no benefit. In reality, the choices which a practice faces are usually between services all of which are effective to an extent, but perhaps some more than others. Should the next addition to the practice team be a counsellor or a homeopath? Is the additional cost of prescribing newer anti-depressants which are selective serotonin re-uptake inhibitors justified? Does a fundholding practice wish to purchase dilatation and curettage as a diagnostic investigation for young women with menorrhagia? Information on effectiveness of treatments is usually patchy at best. But for all of the examples given, there is some information around which could allow the practice to make a more informed choice. A major problem until now has been finding the right information at the right time.

Evidence about effectiveness of treatments has tended to be published piecemeal, scattered across many different medical and scientific journals. It has been difficult even for a conscientious practitioner to make sense of conflicting findings from multiple trials. We are now beginning to see the emergence of digested, up-to-date summaries of evidence on the effectiveness of important treatments. Examples are the series of bulletins *Effective Health Care* which have considered subjects as diverse as the treatment of glue ear, depression in primary care and raised cholesterol levels. Medical journals from time to time publish systematic reviews of the research literature on a particular topic. The Cochrane Centre and the NHS Centre for Reviews and Dissemination are two recent national initiatives dedicated to making more available to health professionals good quality summaries of evidence on the effectiveness of various treatments.

Qualitative approaches

These approaches attempt to capture data about people's preferences and priorities.

What do people want?

There is a very practical reason for having a clear idea of what sort of service people want: it directly influences the extent to which they will make use of it. Even the most effective treatment will be of little use if it is offered in a way which potential users find unacceptable. This may partly explain the low uptake by some ethnic minority groups of services such as cervical screening. Practice staff have frequent opportunities in the course of their daily work to learn about the preferences and opinions of their patients but there will always be gaps in this informal knowledge. It is easiest to find out the preferences of patients who are frequent attenders, articulate and from a similar cultural background to practice staff. It is much more difficult to know what sort of service might be acceptable to people who do not consult very often, who are not registered with the practice, who have language or communication problems or who come from cultural backgrounds with which practice staff are not familiar. There are a variety of ways of getting different angles on the views of current and potential patients which range from the simple use of routinely-available data to quite sophisticated community survey methods:

- *routinely-available markers* (complaints, numbers of patients leaving the practice without changing address)

- *patient surveys* (hand out questionnaire to patients attending the practice, mail questionnaire to registered patients)

- *focus group* (facilitated discussion group to identify and explore issues of interest or concern)

- *rapid appraisal survey* (one-off opinion survey of key members of the local community)

- *community development* (ongoing sampling of local community views and development of services to meet them).

All of these methods have their strengths and weaknesses. The best selection for a particular practice will depend on the question of interest and the resources available to tackle it. The proxy markers, for example, are relatively easy to study because they are already there but focus only on fragments of patients' experience and may be distorted by how easy or difficult patients find it to change practices or use the complaints procedure. A short and simple survey of practice patients can be a good start to identify discrete issues which people feel strongly about, e.g. surgery hours or appointment systems. Box 3.1 shows examples of what two practices in south-east London found when, by different methods, they asked local people what they thought were some of the most important health issues. Note that although all of these are real health issues, only a few of them could be tackled by the practice (or even the NHS) alone. Most would require the support of other agencies such as local government or police. Great achievements are possible with the correct alliances – the Wells Park Health Project was able to persuade the bus company to divert a route through their local housing estate.

The key to a successful needs assessment is to be able to combine these various approaches in a way that will achieve the desired result, within the resources available. An essential prerequisite is to have a clear understanding of why the needs assessment is being undertaken in the first place.

Box 3.1   Examples of what two practices in South-East London found when, by different methods, they asked local people what they thought were some of the most important health issues.

Rapid appraisal
(The Jenner Health Centre)

- Rising crime rate
- Dog mess in streets and parks
- 'Latch key' children returning to empty homes
- Young people who abuse drugs
- Lonely older people

Community development
(The Wells Park Health Project)

- Schoolchildren's health
- Health of Afro-Caribbean people
- Extended services from Wells Park practice
- Poor public transport through a housing estate

4

Information for a primary care-led health service – monitoring performance and quality

Azeem Majeed

The 1991 NHS reforms required family health services authorities to take a more pro-active role in the management of primary health care services. More recently, the move towards a primary care-led NHS and the transfer of resources for purchasing health care from health authorities to fundholding general practices have increased the importance of FHSAs and their successor organizations, the health authorities, holding good information on the practices they administer. As well as having information for needs assessment (see chapter three), information is required to monitor the quality of services provided. Some of the data sources used, plus their drawbacks, are described in Box 4.1. Primary care indicator packages are likely to be produced by many more health authorities in the near future and will become an increasingly important management tool.[1,2] This chapter will describe the variables available in primary care indicator packages and the sources of data from which they are derived, how primary care indicators can be used to investigate differences between practices and their limitations.

Primary care indicator packages

What are they?

Primary care indicators can be divided into broad categories (Box 4.2) and cover areas as diverse as patient characteristics, screening,[3] prescribing, hospital referrals

Box 4.1   Examples of data sources that are used in the production of primary care indicators for general practices.

Data source	Description
Age–sex register	Contains information on all people living in a health authority who are registered with a general practitioner. The information recorded includes age, sex, address, postcode and general practice of each patient. The age–sex register is the most important database used in producing primary care indicators.
	In most health authorities, there are usually more people recorded on the register than actually live in the authority (list inflation). In some areas, the opposite problem may occur (list deflation), that is, fewer patients are present on the age–sex register than actually live in the area. Wrong addresses can also be a problem, especially in inner city areas with high population mobility.
Census data	The 1991 census provides data on demography, ethnicity, housing tenure, employment status and other social factors for geographical areas ranging in size from enumeration districts upwards. An important innovation of the 1991 census was that the census form included a question on the postcode of respondents. This allowed the Office of Population Censuses and Surveys (OPCS) to produce a postcode to enumeration district look-up table which overcomes many of the problems previously encountered in trying to assign postcodes to enumeration districts.
	Problems with census data include the format in which the data is stored, data modification and suppression, sampling error and under-enumeration.
PACT data	PACT (prescribing analysis and cost) data provide information on prescribing for each general practice. The data are available at different levels: total prescribing, British national formulary (BNF) chapter and sections of BNF chapters. The information includes the cost and number of items prescribed for each level of data. PACT data have been enhanced to also include information on individual drugs sometime in 1996.
	Limitations of PACT include: some prescriptions are issued to patients who are not registered with a practice; the number of items per patient is not an ideal measure of the rate of prescribing; and a few patients who are being prescribed very expensive drugs could substantially increase the average prescribing cost per patient for a practice. Finally, If general practitioners increase rates of private prescribing, this will make PACT data less useful.
HES data	HES (hospital episode statistics) data can be used to calculate referral rates by practice down to the level of specialty or

---

Box 4.1 Continued

Data source	Description
	individual diagnosis. HES are often incomplete, the clinical data can be very limited and the accuracy of the data can be poor.
Other health authority data	Other health authority data can be used to provide data on cervical screening and immunization, claims for night visits, staff employed by practices and information on practice character-istics. The main problems with these other sources of data are that they can be inaccurate, are not always computerized and can be difficult to collate.
Data from non-health authority sources	Other data on practices can be obtained from breast screening units (on the uptake of breast screening), community health services (on contacts with their staff), and accident and emer-gency departments (attendance rates at A & E). Mortality data can also be linked with data in age–sex registers to calculate disease specific death rates by practice.

Box 4.2 Examples of primary care indicators for general practices available to health authorities.

Category	Example indicators
Patient data	Demographic breakdown of practice population
	Census derived social variables
Practice characteristics	Number of patients per partner
	Computerization status
	Fundholding status
	Specialist services offered
Target payments	Cervical smear uptake rate
	Percentage of smears that are technically unsuitable
	Immunization uptake
Items of service	Night visiting rate
Prescribing	Prescribing cost per patient
	Percentage of items prescribed generically
	Ratio of inhaled steroids and cromoglycate to bronchodilators
Employed staff	Numbers of categories of employed staff
Hospital referral rates	Referral rates for inpatient care
	Referral rates for outpatient care

---

and practice staffing. Many indicators are produced by using data from two different sources. For example, census-derived variables can be produced for general prac-tices by linking the postcodes of patients on health authority age–sex registers with census data for enumeration districts.[4] Figure 4.1 shows the distribution of one such

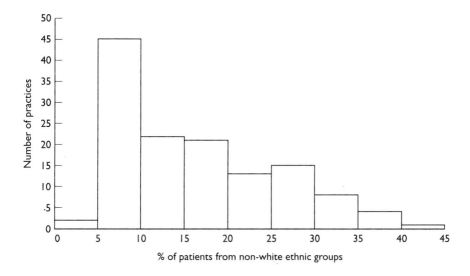

Figure 4.1 Distribution of expected percentage of patients from non-white ethnic groups in 131 general practices in Merton, Sutton and Wandsworth.

census-derived variable, the expected percentage of the practice population from non-white ethnic groups, in 131 general practices in Merton, Sutton and Wandsworth Health Authority. The expected percentage of non-white patients varies ten-fold across the practices, from 4% to just over 40%.

How can they be used?

This kind of information on practices is useful in planning and monitoring services. For example, health authorities could use the information to help them plan services based in primary care for the management of haemoglobinopathies such as sickle cell disease and thalassaemia. Health authorities can also compare the social and ethnic characteristics of practice populations against the utilization of health services.[5] In Figure 4.2, the information on the percentage of practice population from non-white ethnic groups is plotted against the cervical smear uptake rates for the same practices. As the figure shows, there is a strong negative association between uptake rates and the estimated percentage of people from non-white ethnic groups. However, despite this association, some practices in areas with large numbers of people from ethnic minorities achieved high cervical smear uptake rates. Further study of such practices may lead to the identification of methods that can be used to increase uptake rates in such areas.

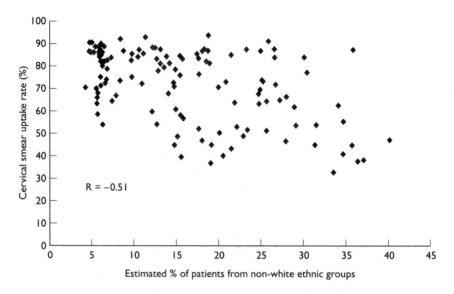

Figure 4.2 Scatterplot of cervical smear uptake rates against estimated percentage of the practice population from non-white ethnic groups in 131 general practices in Merton, Sutton and Wandsworth.

For allocating resources

By collating information on practices in one readily accessible source, primary care indicators for general practices will allow health authorities to monitor more easily the performance of practices, and therefore allocate resources to practices for staff, premises, hospital referrals and prescribing on a rational basis. Because general practices have been funded on the basis of previous spending, there is potential for the resources available for primary care services to be distributed inequitably. By comparing the resources allocated to practices with measures of need (see chapter three), health authorities can attempt to ensure that resources are allocated more fairly to general practices. For example, they can use primary care indicators to help ensure that fundholding practices receive similar funding to non-fundholding practices.

The development of league tables

Primary care indicators will allow health authorities to rank practices and therefore produce league tables of practice performance; a development which many general practitioners will find threatening. This approach could be applied to cervical smear and immunization uptake rates, and the percentage of drugs prescribed generically. General practitioners who work in deprived communities where social problems and population mobility are both high, may feel that such league tables will unfairly label them as 'poor-performing' practices.

Comparing like with like

Health authorities therefore need to ensure that any league tables they produce are interpreted appropriately; primary care medical advisers and public health physicians will both have a role in doing this. One method of taking social factors into account when assessing a practice's performance is to use the primary care indicators to calculate expected values for a practice based on the characteristics of the population it serves and to compare these expected values with the actual value obtained by the practice. For example, in March 1994 cervical smear uptake rates in the general practices in Merton, Sutton and Wandsworth varied from 33% to 95%, a three-fold variation.[6] Box 4.3 shows the results of a multiple regression

---

Box 4.3 Forwards stepwise regression model of cervical smear uptake rates on patient and practice characteristics for 131 general practices in Merton, Sutton and Wandsworth.

Variable	Regression coefficient	P value
Intercept	66.6	<0.0001
Ethnic minority	−0.53	0.0003
Number of partners	2.05	0.01
Under-fives	1.35	0.02
Female partner*	6.28	0.01
Computer*	5.64	0.02
List inflation	−0.45	0.02

* present = 1, absent = 0

Cervical smear uptake rates in the 131 general practices in Merton, Sutton and Wandsworth varied from 33% to 95% in March 1994. Entering the primary care indicators as dependent variables and cervical smear uptake rate as the independent variable into a forwards stepwise regression model with an entry criterion of P = 0.05 resulted in a multiple correlation coefficient of 0.73 with six indicators explaining 53% of the variation in cervical smear uptake rates. The number of partners in a practice and the percentage of the practice population under five years of age were both positive predictors of uptake rates. For example, an increase of one in the number of partners resulted in an increase of about 2% in the predicted uptake rate for a practice. Rates were also 6.28% higher in practices with a female partner than in those without and 5.64% higher in computerized practices than in non-computerized practices, after adjusting for other factors. For each increase of 1% in the percentage of the practice population under five years of age the predicted uptake rate for a practice would increase by 1.35%. The estimated percentage of the practice population from ethnic minority groups and the estimated list inflation for a practice were both negative predictors of cervical smear uptake rates. For example, for each 1% increase in the ethnic variable and in list inflation, the predicted smear uptake rate for a practice decreased by 0.53% and 0.45% respectively. The results of the regression analysis raised several interesting hypotheses that could be tested in further research. For example, could the introduction of female general practitioners into inner city general practices increase cervical smear uptake rates?

Box 4.4 Observed and predicted cervical smear uptake rates, and difference between them, for eight practices in Merton, Sutton and Wandsworth.

Practice	Cervical smear uptake rate (ranking)	Predicted smear uptake rate	Actual–predicted (ranking)
A	77.0 (66)	47.3	29.7 (1)
B	87.2 (18)	60.4	26.8 (2)
C	55.2 (105)	53.5	1.7 (60)
D	46.6 (119)	45.5	1.1 (65)
E	88.2 (14)	88.0	0.2 (67)
F	85.3 (34)	85.6	−0.3 (68)
G	48.8 (115)	74.0	−25.2 (130)
H	44.8 (122)	71.2	−26.4 (131)

Source: Regression model shown in Box 4.3.

General practitioners who work in deprived communities where social problems and population mobility are both high, may feel that league tables of practice performance will unfairly label them as 'poor-performing' practices. Health authorities must therefore ensure that any league tables they produce are interpreted appropriately. It is possible to produce 'adjusted' performance measures, and these adjusted measures are likely to be fairer than unadjusted measures that do not take account of social, ethnic or demographic factors. For example, using the types of census derived variables that are contained in many primary care indicator packages, cervical smear uptake rates can be adjusted to take into account the characteristics of the populations that practices serve. The table above illustrates this by using data from the regression model shown in Box 4.3 for eight practices with varying levels of cervical smear coverage. As the table shows, the rankings of practices can alter markedly when patient and practice characteristics are taken into account. The performance of both Practice A and Practice B appears much better when adjusted for patient and practice factors, whereas the performance of Practice G and Practice H appears much worse. An alternative approach to producing adjusted measures of performance would be to only adjust for patient characteristics. Further discussion would be required between general practitioners and health authorities to determine which approach is more appropriate.

analysis of the uptake rates achieved by these practices. Patient and practice variables from a locally developed primary care indicator package explained 53% of the variation in uptake rates. Using the results of this analysis, an expected cervical smear uptake rate for each practice was calculated and then compared with the actual uptake rate achieved by the practice; the results are shown for eight practices in Box 4.4. As shown, the rankings of practices can alter markedly when patient and practice characteristics are taken into account. The performance of both Practice A and Practice B appears much better when adjusted for patient and practice factors, whereas the performance of Practice G and Practice H appears much worse.

Resource allocation

Some health authorities may wish to use league tables to identify and reward high performing practices by increasing the resources allocated to them for staff and premises. Conversely, if measures of health need are used to redirect resources into areas with a high need for health care, then less well developed practices (which are usually located in such areas) may receive more resources. Because such practices may not have the capacity to utilize additional resources effectively, this may have a demotivating effect on the morale of the more innovative practices which are not benefiting from additional resources. The uncritical application of primary care indicators in the allocation of resources should therefore be avoided.

Clinical audit

As well as the benefits they offer to health authorities, primary care indicators also offer benefits to general practitioners. They can be used to identify areas in which a practice deviates from the norm and thus serve as the basis of clinical and administrative audit. For example, a practice with a high night visiting rate or a low rate of generic prescribing may wish to investigate this further. These types of audits can also highlight potential problems or limitations of routinely collected data.

A practical example

In one such investigation, the Sefton Medical Audit Advisory Group identified a potential problem with the coding of inadequate smears on the standard cervical cytology form HMR101/5/C. The coding on the form does not allow smears that are inadequate because of the poor technique of the person taking the smear (for example, because they are scanty, air dried or from the wrong part of the cervix) to be distinguished from smears that are unsuitable for reasons not linked with the technique of the person taking the smear (for example, because they are blood-stained or obscured by polymorphs). This reduces the usefulness of the primary care indicator 'percentage of smears that are technically inadequate'. The Sefton Medical Audit Group and the Sefton Cytology Group have written to the Department of Health asking them to address this issue.

Practice quality initiatives

Primary care indicators can also help practices to identify areas which are priorities for improvement, and help them to monitor their performance over time. The indicators therefore have a role in practice-based quality improvement programmes. To facilitate the use of primary care indicators in this way, health authorities should plan and introduce their primary care indicator packages only after consultation and negotiation with local general practitioners. This will help ensure that general practitioners find the packages and the variables they contain useful in their day-to-day work and in the management of their own practices.

Research and development

Finally, primary care indicators demonstrate the extent of variation in many aspects of general practice and can be used as the basis of descriptive research into medical practice variations in primary care. Baker and Klein[1] showed how primary care indicators could be used to investigate differences between family health services authorities. A similar approach can be used to investigate differences between practices, and this has been done in the areas of cervical cancer screening, breast cancer screening, night visiting and prescribing.

What are the problems?

Quantity not quality

Primary care indicators do have limitations, the most important of which is that they only measure certain aspects of practice performance. For example, they can tell us what a practice's referral rate is but tell us nothing about the appropriateness or quality of these referrals. Primary care indicators also tell us nothing about what most general practitioners would consider to be their most important role, the clinical care of the individual patient.

Perverse incentives

There is a risk that primary care indicators will create perverse incentives for general practitioners in that they will concentrate on improving the indicators rather than improving the quality of care they provide to their patients. For example, a high ratio of inhaled steroids and cromoglycate to inhaled bronchodilators is considered to be an indicator of good prescribing for asthma. A practice with a low ratio could indiscriminately increase its prescribing of steroids and cromoglycate to improve the ratio without ensuring that any additional prescribing is appropriate or that other aspects of care – such as patient education – are improved.

Rubbish in, rubbish out

Primary care indicators are constructed from routine data; there are many errors in such data, especially in age–sex registers (list inflation), census data (under-enumeration) and referrals data (inaccurate and incomplete coding). Finally, indicators on prescribing are derived from prescribing analyses and cost (PACT) data; with the steadily increasing cost of NHS prescriptions it is likely that more drugs will either be prescribed on private prescriptions (which are not recorded on PACT) or bought over the counter, making less accurate prescribing indicators derived from PACT data. Health authorities need to be aware of the limitations of primary care indicators, and should not use them uncritically when they assess the performance of general practitioners.

Who should use them?

Indicators about health authorities and NHS trusts are made available to a wide audience, including journalists and the public. Should primary care indicators about general practices be published and made available to the public in the same way? One of the aims of the 1990 general practitioner contract was to increase patient choice and encourage patients to register with practices that offered high-quality services. Patients do have access to a limited amount of information on practices (for example, in practices' leaflets and in the directory of practices held by health authorities). However, most patients choose a practice either because of its location or because it has been recommended by a friend or neighbour. If patients are to be encouraged to choose their general practitioner more objectively, then they will require better data on the performance of their local general practices and on the services that they offer. Some health authorities may therefore wish to place primary care indicators in the public domain. Although some general practitioners may oppose the publication of primary care indicators, we already have league tables for schools and hospitals, and the publication of league tables for general practices may therefore be inevitable. However, in view of the controversy raised by league tables for schools and hospitals, and the lack of consensus between general practitioners and managers over what constitutes 'good' performance (for example, is cheap prescribing good or bad?), this is a development that health authorities should handle with great sensitivity. However, where general practitioners have been consulted about primary care indicators before their release, they have generally been well received and have been found useful. Even if they are not released widely, health authorities are likely to make much greater use of primary care indicators as part of their new role in monitoring and developing general practice. They should therefore collaborate with general practitioners to improve the quality of data on which primary care indicators are based; and start to discuss with their local general practices how they propose to use primary care indicators in the management of primary care services. Finally, managers, public health physicians and general practitioners must remember that although primary care indicators have many uses, they are only one of the many tools that need to be used to improve the quality of primary care services.

Reference

1   Baker D, Klein R. (1991) Explaining outputs of primary care: population and practice factors. *British Medical Journal.* **303**: 225–9.

2   Hanlon A, Hargreaves S. (1994) Performance indicators for general practice. *Journal of Epidemiology and Community Health.* **48**: 502.

3   Majeed FA, Cook DG, Given-Wilson R *et al.* (1995) Do general practitioners influence the uptake of breast cancer screening? *Journal of Medical Screening.* **2**: 119–24.

4   Majeed FA, Cook DG, Polonieki J *et al.* (1995) Sociodemographic variables for general practices: use of census data. *British Medical Journal.* **310**: 1373–4.

5   Majeed FA, Cook DG, Hilton S *et al.* (1995) Annual night visiting rates in 129 general practices in one family health services authority: association with patient and general practice characteristics. *British Journal of General Practice.* **45**: 531–5.

6   Majeed FA, Cook DG, Anderson HR *et al.* (1994) Using patient and general practice characteristics to explain variations in cervical smear uptake rates. *British Medical Journal.* **308**: 1272–6.

5

Stimulus for change – the evolution of fundholding

Howard Freeman

*Fundholding has travelled a long distance since the first three hundred prac-
tices tentatively stepped out on the journey in April 1991. What was allegedly
an afterthought tacked on to the NHS reforms has shown itself to be a
veritable jewel in the crown. The origin of the road fundholders are following
goes back to Mrs Thatcher's cavalierly announced review of the health service
in 1987. Alan Maynard, Professor of Health Economics at York University, at
a seminar organized by the Office of Health Economics gave a presentation
based on the American health maintenance organizations' concept of giving
general practitioners the capacity to buy hospital services on behalf of their
patients. The American economist Enthoven who, of course, was a very
powerful advocate of competition in the health service, was asked to come
to Britain to comment on the NHS. His views, the views of Maynard, the
views of those advocating insurance-based schemes, such as Oliver Letwin,
and reviews published by Dr Michael Goldsmith and David Willetts in a
pamphlet from the Centre of Policy Studies were all distilled together to form
the basis of the fundholding scheme.[1]*

Historical background

Small beginnings

Initially the scheme was limited to practices or groups of practices covering 9000
patients or more. This was intended to minimize the random risk of budgets.
However, in order to run a practice of 9000 patients or more a practice needs to
have a well-developed management structure, which undoubtedly helps in entering
fundholding.

The scheme initially had three elements for which the practices had responsibility. From the mid-1960s GPs had an element of their support staff costs reimbursed from Family Health Service Authorities. Normally they would expect to get 70% of the cost returned. For fundholders this became a real cash allocation and they were freed from many of the petty restrictions around seeking authorization for changes in staffing structure and postholders. For the first time the open-ended and demand-led practice prescribing budgets were cash limited in fundholding practices. Again notional cost was converted into actual cash amounts for fundholders.

The final area fundholders could purchase was initially limited to hospital outpatient services, diagnostic services which included pathology and radiology, open access services and a restricted range of elective surgical procedures. Although this did, for many, appear to be quite a wide range it quickly became apparent that it was in fact far too restrictive.

Shifting the power base

It was perhaps one of the unfortunate coincidences for the NHS reforms that the launch of the exciting concept of fundholding coincided with the acrimony of the imposition of the 1990 Contract for General Practice. For many general practitioners the purchaser/provider separation, GP fundholding and the 1990 Contract all got blurred in a mist of anger and despair. For a few with perhaps a greater clarity of vision it was absolutely apparent that one of the key points about fundholding was that it had the potential to reverse the whole power balance in the NHS and it would be surprising if that point was lost to the consultant-led leadership of the British Medical Association who opposed the scheme.

Community not consultant needs?

From the outset of the NHS, developments in the service were determined purely by the wishes of hospital consultants. These reflected their own interests, aspirations and desires but most certainly did not reflect the needs or wishes of the communities in which they were based. Increasingly this led to a mis-match in provision and demand which perhaps is seen nowhere better than in the secondary service provision and the relative lack of primary care provision in London. General management in the 1980s was thought to be the solution to this but except in a few places general managers were unable to affect significantly the direction of travel or services.

Linking clinical decision-making and budgetary control

Fundholding had the benefit of taking the money necessary for the service out of the often far too cosy relationships between managers and hospital clinicians and putting it into the hands of community-based fellow professionals who could counter spurious professional claims. Even more powerful is the fact that GPs have had long experience at running their own business and understand the value of money perhaps far more than colleagues in the hospital service did. What you now had for the first time was a lever sufficiently powerful to move the vested hospital interest. It is perhaps, therefore, not surprising that if you look at the 300 practices who became the first wave of fundholders you see a disproportionate percentage of practices represented who had a great deal of experience in both local and national medical politics.

Allocating resources

Anyone who reads the documentation published by the Department of Health in the early days of the scheme will be left in little doubt that it was always the intention that ultimately fundholders would be funded by some form of weighted capitation formula. Such a formula was not available for the early waves of fundholders and the only way budgets could be set was by an attempt to cost historical activity. This was clearly unsatisfactory for several reasons.

Poor information

In most places there was little idea of what previous historical activity was. The practices themselves collected very accurate information. Information available from hospital systems was usually wildly inaccurate if present at all. This led to many heated arguments. Coupled with this was the pricing structure from the provider units. Because of the poor information databases they had and because of the instruction that price should equal cost and the whole message of steady state for the early days, much of the pricing could at best be described as a finger in the wind. Fundholders realized quite early on that in terms of information they had the upper hand and there was little doubt at all that in many places budgets were set in the fundholders' favour. However, in many other places, due to all the inaccuracies, fundholders did not gain but lost; there is no evidence whatsoever that there was any policy to deliberately overfund fundholders in the early years. Nevertheless many were quick to argue that fundholders in fact were not better purchasers than their health authority counterparts but were merely more generously funded, and that is a debate which is still continuing.

Profits?

Probably one of the most controversial parts of the scheme is the whole concept of overspends and underspends on budget. If fundholders, after the end of the financial year audit, have money left from any of the heads of their budget, that money can then be spent in a wide variety of ways for the benefit of the patients of their practice. They can use it to purchase more of the procedures within the fundholding list, they can use it to purchase equipment to use in the practice and perhaps most controversially they can use it to extend their premises. It cannot be used at present to purchase new premises and it must be stressed that there is total separation between the practice profit and loss account and the fundholding account. Nevertheless if any part of the underspend is used to purchase a capital asset, in subsequent years this asset can be sold on to incoming partners and be converted into a real profit. This however should be viewed from the perspective of how GPs prior to fundholding were able to finance premises. This was through interest-free cost rents, and improvement grants (up to 90% in inner London) which could be sold on to incoming partners to make a real profit. They can also receive a year-on-year rent from their authority on these premises. From this perspective the argument about the use of fundholder savings is really a non-event.

Losses

What is of more concern is the issue of overspends. If a fundholder overspends their budget then that overspend becomes a charge on their health authority. Specifically it is not top-sliced from their next year's budget nor does it become a charge on any savings they have accrued. In addition, in order to minimize the random risk and help prevent the so-called cherry picking of only well patients, there is a stop loss limit initially set at £5000 and now increased to £6000 per patient for hospital services in each year. Anything above this again becomes a charge to the district health authority. Many would argue that this really is inequitable. Most fundholders would be happy to assume their own risk but the trade off would have to be more than a one year budgeting system; perhaps three year rolling budgets, which at present the Treasury is reluctant to accept.

The growth of fundholding

Despite continuing professional and political opposition from the Labour Party fundholding has grown substantially year-on-year (Table 5.1). The Conservative win in the 1992 election was clearly a major factor in this as it became quite clear that the policy would certainly continue for the life of the government. In 1993 the scheme was extended to include health visiting and district nursing services, services for people with learning disabilities, chiropody and dietetics as well as community mental health services. The minimum list size required to enter the scheme has been lowered from 9000 through to 7000 and down to 5000 from 1 April 1996. Although this has enabled more practices to be eligible to enter the scheme and

Table 5.1 Percentage of population (England) covered by GP fundholding.

1991/92	1992/93	1993/94	1994/95	1995/96	1996/97
7%	13%	25%	35%	41%	53% projected

has undoubtedly led in part to the increase in the scheme, there is no doubt the smaller the practice size the greater the variation in need and the associated variation in expenditure.

Risk of small practices

A study by Crump et al.[7] showed that the year-on-year variation on annual expenditure around the mean could be 15% for a large practice (24 000 patients), and this almost doubled to 27.5% for a small practice (9000 patients). Reducing the list size increases the level of financial risk, i.e. increases the probability of overspends and underspends because any single event has a more pronounced impact. However, this risk can be reduced by expanding the scope of the scheme as the probability of a given practice exceeding its budget is reduced. It can be argued that increasing the number of elements in the scheme reduces the random risk in a way analogous to having a portfolio of shares. It is therefore not surprising that in conjunction with the fall of the list size to 5000 from 1 April 1996 the scheme has been further expanded to include more elements of community nursing services as well as further elements of elective surgery.

Community fundholding

As well as the changes in what is now called standard fundholding, as a consequence of a series of road shows attended by the former Minister of Health, Dr Brian Mawhinney, it was clear that many GPs were interested in a model of fundholding where they would have to be responsible for fewer elements of services. Many GPs were saying they wished to be responsible for their staff budgets and their prescribing budgets, but would also wish to be responsible for purchasing community nursing services, diagnostic services and outpatient services. This became the precursor of the Community Fundholding Scheme. Unfortunately providers were reluctant to allow outpatient services to be included within this scheme. Most providers had very poor outpatient information systems and outpatients were poorly costed. Providers argued that it would push up transaction costs tremendously if they had to differentiate yet another level of purchasers. This was unfortunate as there was little doubt at all that one of the areas GP fundholders have most significantly influenced has been outpatient services. Nearly all fundholders have sought to control the plague of unnecessary repeat follow-up in outpatients as well as the nonsense of new referrals being seen by a doctor often more junior than the GP. From outpatient budgets have come some of the most substantial savings to fundholders. However, the provider argument won the day and the new community fundholding scheme launched on 1 April 1996 only has diagnostic and open access elements from the hospitals. It will however be open to fundholding practices with list sizes as low as 3000 patients as there is little random risk here, although probably little scope for making real savings except from prescribing budgets.

Multi-funding

One of the most interesting spin-offs from the scheme has undoubtedly been the concept of multifunds. From its outset the scheme enabled groups of practices to come together to form a single fund unit if that was necessary to make up the minimum number criteria. In the early days very few of these happened. The history of general practice has always been one of isolation with very little joint and cooperative working between neighbouring practices. If one looks at the situation in the inner city of London, one actually sees large numbers of very small practices very close together in a highly competitive situation and it becomes quite obvious why joint working as originally envisaged did not occur. A milestone down the road was the decision by nearly all the practices in the London Boroughs of Kingston and Richmond to set up a central joint purchasing structure to enable them to enter the fundholding scheme in a more collaborative and co-operative fashion. Initially this was called a superfund but rapidly became a multifund and the name has stuck.

Who can best purchase health care?

Fundholding at its outset was a rural and shire counties sport. Very few inner city practices either had sufficient patients to enter the scheme or were not well organized or motivated enough so to do. Many health authorities were far from supportive of fundholding. From the financial model they saw fundholders taking their resources and by limiting the amount of cash they had so increasing their own random risk. Fundholders were no respecters of cosy sweetheart relationships between providers and purchasers and were quite happy to upset apple carts. It became quite apparent that fundholders understood the purchasing function much better than many health authorities and could do it far better. Health authorities were not best pleased to have ministers berating them for their inability to purchase as well as fundholders.

Competitive purchasing

Many health authorities had no experience of working with general practitioners and had no respect for their abilities. They did not understand or agree with the political concepts behind fundholding and were often profoundly antagonistic towards fundholders. It was said that the term co-purchasers was actually short for competitive purchasers rather than anything else. Fundholders were perceived by health authorities to enjoy freedoms unheard of by them and as daily they were deluged with more instructions and restrictions so they became increasingly envious of the freedom fundholders appeared to enjoy. Many set up quasi commissioning groups in an attempt to persuade GPs that they would be responsive to their needs through that route and that there was no need for them to enter the fundholding scheme. By the mid-1990s GPs had begun to see through these schemes.

Many of them had been set up in inner city areas and it was thought unlikely that these practices would ever be able to enter the fundholding scheme. As a consequence of their frustration at the failure of locality purchasing schemes many inner city GPs began to beat a path to Kingston and Richmond to look at the way their multifund worked. Multifunds began to mushroom. Whilst there are many variations on the theme and every multifund believes it has solved the problem of purchasing, the basis of all multifunds is that groups of practices join together to form single fund units for statutory purposes and collectively pay towards the multifund structure which does a variable amount of the purchasing, contract monitoring, financial monitoring and other requirements of the scheme for them. But what is of great interest is the added value of multifunds. Whilst initially the practices only joined together to purchase they inexorably get drawn into greater areas of co-working and joint planning. Multifunds are in fact an agent of improving the delivery of primary care, often quite poor in some of these practices, as well as beginning to draw out isolated GPs into a more collaborative framework.

Accountability

As more GPs entered fundholding so it became clear that there would have to be formalization of how fundholders related to other parts of the NHS and how they were to be held accountable, not just in providing terms but in terms of delivering national and local priorities. Nobody was unhappy with the concept, the problem was how to deliver it. In many places relationships between fundholders and health authorities were at an all time low. Whilst most FHSAs were supportive of fundholders, fundholders were seeing FHSA staff being culled as part of the merger between the two authorities and beginning to find often authoritative and dictatorial health authority staff replacing facilitative FHSA staff. Such was the climate that the Accountability Framework for Fundholders was launched in 1995.[3]

National guidance

The accountability framework was an attempt to tread a middle path. It clearly set out the responsibilities and accountabilities of fundholders but made it clear that there was to be no heavy handed management of this by the health authorities. The accountability framework needed to be read in conjunction with an executive letter published in November 1994 (EL(94)79), *Towards a primary care-led NHS*. There is little doubt that the key influence to the writing of this document has been the success of GP fundholding. Whatever they say now it is doubtful if anyone in 1990 envisaged that this document could possibly have been published by 1994.

Unevaluated – but still the way forward

The major criticism of fundholding is that it has been unevaluated. This executive letter is the evaluation and the statement of the success of the scheme. It is the key to where health services in this country are going. It signals unequivocally the intended shift in emphasis towards a primary care-led NHS and primary care-led purchasing. It signals that increasingly decisions about health services will be taken within the context of, and informed by, the perspective of primary care. Critical and pivotal in the success of this is GP fundholding. The delivery of this vision depends principally on action at local level and that will be by partnerships between providers and health authorities and with fundholding GPs at its centre.

What has fundholding achieved?

Whilst fundholding has undeniably not been formally unevaluated no one can deny it has been responsible for two major changes. Firstly shifts in health services from secondary to primary care fundholders have made major advances in shifting work out of the hospital sector into a primary care setting. In the main that setting has been their own practice and many would argue they have done this gratis to the NHS. It will not be until we have clearly defined what comprises general medical services that we can actually see the extent that fundholders have made this shift. But nevertheless this shift has been made and inherent within the concept of the primary care-led NHS is the presumption in favour of supporting people at home, all in their own community, unless their needs can be more appropriately and effectively met in hospitals.

Bespoke purchasing

The second clear change attributable to fundholding has been that truly in fundholding-based purchasing the money does follow the patient. Health authorities are still locked into large contracts which are not sensitive to individual patient needs. The early work done by Glenister et al.[5] clearly shows that fundholders have moved very rapidly to contracting around the individual patient. They provide a bespoke service to fit the needs of that individual patient and are able to do this because they have not precommitted their cash into large contracts. Whilst this is unquestionably better for the individual patient it is of course a much more risky way of contracting for the providers and there is no doubt at all that it increases transaction costs for providers. Nevertheless many of the American health maintenance organizations pride themselves on how low they can keep transaction costs and we should be looking at why British transaction costs cannot be kept down in the same manner as those of the best in the United States.

The future of fundholding

What of the future for fundholding? Unfortunately it is still caught up in the political rhetoric between the two major parties. Despite the repeatedly avowed intention of the Labour Party to abolish fundholding should it hold office after the next election, it seems inconceivable that the same party which openly admits it cannot turn the clock back in the health service would or could achieve this. Whether genuine or not, there appears to be a view held by the Labour Party that most fundholders were not willing recruits but pressed converts. There can be little doubt that some authorities did put undue pressure on some GPs to become fundholders. But these must be the minority not the majority. The most telling point is always how few GPs, once in the scheme, have wished to leave it. Having pushed through this major cultural change in the NHS, would it be possible or credible to reverse it? Most believe the answer to this is no and that all one would see should there be a change of government is some form of rebadging of the scheme with some minor changes in accountability and the use of savings.

Spectrum

If we accept that there will be different models of practice-based purchasing then we must perceive a spectrum. This spectrum will range from those practices who merely wish to give advice to a health authority who will continue to purchase all services on their behalf, through the different types of fundholding to total purchasing.

Total purchasing

Total purchasing was announced as part of the executive letter, *Towards a primary care-led NHS*. The best definition of total purchasing is to extend to GP purchasers the ability to purchase and commission the whole range of services which currently a health authority can. Initially 25 pilots were to be announced with a full evaluation but the demand to be one of the first pilots was so overwhelming that the numbers were increased so that 52 pilots were ultimately announced, leaving about five times that number of practices disappointed. These pilots range from single practices right up to pilots which cover populations of 100 000. There is very little framework around the pilots and most believe that the best and the worst ideas from each will in some way be distilled to give us a better understanding of the way total purchasing works.

Total purchasing should enable us to ensure a more equitable distribution of funds at practice levels. As health authorities' allocations become more formula driven, the disparity between that and the lack of a formula for standard fundholding will become more apparent. It should be possible to devise a formula for allocating down to total purchasing pilots, which whilst not identical with that of the allocation basis to health authorities, is at least compatible with it. Clearly the evaluation will have to look at whether it is feasible for GPs to purchase all services both in terms of the time element and the risk element involved. It can be argued that there are some services which are not really commissioned at all by health authorities but are in fact paid for by them but driven by others. A good example of this would be issues around forensic psychiatry and court decisions. We may well arrive at a scenario where practice-based total purchasing will only be responsible for some areas and other areas such as those mentioned previously will be purchased perhaps by large, population-based alternative purchasers.

Personal versus public health

Will total purchasing practices be able to purchase with the same individual sensitivity as they currently do for fundholding? If they do manage to move from large contracts to more individually-based contracts, will providers be able to cope with both the transaction implications and the risk of this? Purchasing a whole range of services on behalf of small populations may well enable more sensitive purchasing around individuals, but can this be equated with the needs of larger populations which the good health authority purchasers are beginning to come to terms with? How will public health integrate with both the top-down approach of health authority purchasers and the bottom-up perspective of total purchasing pilots? Finally if we have practices responsible for purchasing the whole spectrum of secondary care and wishing to make substantial shifts from the secondary to the primary sector, what will happen to the contractual basis for the delivery of general practice? Clearly the 1990 contract will fall apart at the seams but equally we will have to look at a much more stringent regulatory framework, both around their accreditation for delivering an extended range of primary care services and for their actual ability to deliver.

A practical way forward

By posing these questions perhaps we can come to one model of future relationships between the health authorities and general practice. Figure 5.1 begins to show this relationship. We know that the new health authorities will have very clear roles in developing local strategy and ensuring both local and national strategies are delivered. They will have a role in supporting practices in both the delivery of primary care and their purchasing role, whether that be direct purchasing or through the commissioning route. They will also have a regulatory role, initially regulating fundholders and probably total purchasing practices, but the accountability framework begins to spell out that perhaps there will be a regulatory role around commissioning practices as well. They will inherit from the FHSAs the responsibility to plan and supervise the delivery of general practice and it will not be a great step to turn that into a regulatory role for general practice. Many are already beginning to let contracts for an extended range of primary care services and once the definition of core general medical services is defined then clearly this will become an easier role.

Competitive purchasing

What of the health authority purchasing function? If we assume that the future roles of the health authority are, broadly speaking, regulatory then does the purchasing

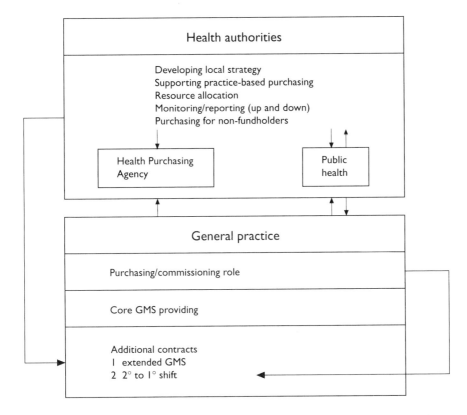

Figure 5.1 Model of future relationship between health authorities and general practice.

role have to be within the statutory local organization? Some purchasing, e.g. old regional specialties already occur non-locally through lead purchasing. One could well envisage a market in different purchasers. Similarly health authorities, fund-holders and total purchasers will all need input from public health. This could be 'purchased' by all these different purchasers depending on their requirements. If one pursues this model further then one can look at the private purchase of health care and wonder perhaps if this is not a market they would wish to enter.

Conclusions

This chapter has tried to take you through the evolution of practice-based purchasing. We are still in a very rapid evolutionary phase and whether the final outcome will be part of the mainstream of the development of health services or merely a sub-branch we do not yet know. The whole of this needs to be viewed from a context of the debate we are beginning to enter about prioritization and rationing in the context of a finite financial resource. None of this is incompatible with the concept of a National Health Service. Throughout its history the National Health Service has been an evolving concept, the only clearly sacrosanct ethos behind it being care universally available and free at the point of delivery, which is fully compatible with fundholding.

References

1 Butler J. (1992) *Patients, policies and politics: before and after Working for Patients.* Open University Press, Milton Keynes.

2 Crump BJ, Gibbon JE, Drummond MF et al. (1991) Fundholding in General Practice and Financial Risk. *British Medical Journal.* **302**: 1582–4.

3 NHS Executive. (1995) Accountability framework for GP fundholders. *EL(95)54.*

4 NHS Executive. (1994) Developing NHS purchasing and GP fundholding. Towards a primary care-led NHS. *EL(94)79.*

5 Glennister H, Matsaganis N, Owens P et al. (1994) *Implementing GP Fundholding – Wild Card or Winning Hand.* Open University Press, Milton Keynes.

6

Commissioning –
the best for all

Andrew Willis

The development of GP commissioning is a remarkable story of success. It is an approach to the 1990 changes in the NHS that has been developed largely by GPs themselves. It is one that ensures greater influence for GPs in planning the services required for their patients while preserving the fundamental principles of the NHS. It produces beneficial results for relatively little effort and it is fair to patients and practices. At the same time it also ensures that accountability for fiscal constraint in NHS resources remains where it belongs, with the government.

What is commissioning?

In implementing the 1990 NHS reforms a fundamental error is made by almost all policy makers when they fail to appreciate the difference between planning and procurement, between commissioning and purchasing. Commissioning is largely a strategic exercise. It may be defined as 'the process of gathering and analysing the wants and needs of a population, and identifying the services required to meet those needs. It includes monitoring those services as they are delivered'. The setting of priorities is an inherent component of commissioning. Purchasing, however, is an operational task; 'the interpretation of commissioning plans and the construction and implementation of time-related purchasing plans'. Rationing, the deliberate constraint of access to services, is an inevitability of purchasing.

   Most GPs will feel it appropriate to contribute to commissioning but see rationing as something outside their role as a family doctor. All GPs, fundholders and non-fundholders together, should be encouraged to take part in commissioning and supported in that endeavour. It is a task common to both. The only fundamental difference between them is in their choice of purchaser. It is of greater importance to the NHS that a practice contributes constructively to a co-ordinated commissioning exercise than that it is a direct purchaser, yet current incentives exactly invert those priorities.

There are nearly 100 commissioning groups working throughout the UK, from the Highlands to the south coast, from East Anglia to Northern Ireland. About half involve fundholders directly or indirectly and a reasonable estimate of the number of patients involved is 15 million. The many attractions of commissioning for patients, GPs and the NHS are summarized in Box 6.1.

Box 6.1 Benefits of GP commissioning.

- Cohesive development of local strategy and services

- Adherence to the fundamental principles of the NHS

- Equity of access for patients according to clinical need

- Equality of opportunity for practices

- Economy of effort

- Maintenance of statutory accountability

How to do it – the principles

So how may GPs be involved appropriately in developing the NHS? Four criteria can be used to assess the suitability of different approaches:

1   commissioning and purchasing should be integrated at district, locality and practice levels, using appropriate populations for different services

2   primary and secondary care clinicians should be encouraged to work together to make effective use of the available resources to provide high quality services

3   equity of access according to clinical need should be assured within appropriately sized populations for different services

4   equality of opportunity and resources should be available for all practices that wish to contribute to the development of their local services.

Only approaches that meet these four criteria have a place in the development of a health service that remains true to its core principles. GP commissioning is one.

Basic requirements

Enthusiasm

A health authority needs to be enthusiastic about developing commissioning, at liberty to do so, and with resources available to support the exercise.

The need for true partnership

Few health authorities yet understand what is required of them to make GP commissioning effective. First and foremost there is a need for a written, working partnership between the health authority and a representative group of GPs which has a mandate to give opinion, and make decisions, on behalf of the practices it represents.

The need for resources

If GPs are to work in partnership with the DHA then resources must be made available to establish, support and sustain that relationship. While this should take place locally it requires endorsement and encouragement from the NHS Executive.

The need for information

There is a need for appropriate systems to be established that allow the integrated collection, collation and dissemination of the information required to establish the wants and needs of populations from individual practice size through localities to the district. The health authority and public health physicians have key roles here, and there is a need for financial support to be made available equally to fundholders and non-fundholders for their computer costs.

Representation of all practices

Commissioning is an inclusive, collaborative approach. It needs a managed market economy based upon collective benefit rather than one which is exclusive and acquisitive, based primarily on self-interest. There is a need for a core group of GPs that has a mandate to represent all practices within the locality, district or both.

Working together

In its entirety commissioning should be a multi-disciplinary exercise concerning a given population, involving representatives of patients' opinions as well as the health and social care professions. The concept of a primary care-led NHS is not synonymous with a GP-led one. In essence this suggests sub-district populations (localities), each with some form of co-ordinating group containing appropriate representation from primary care (fundholders and non-fundholders together), the health authority, social services and other local voices.

Communication

Locality co-ordinating groups are important bodies, offering cohesive planning at the same time as sensitivity to the needs of local communities. They draw up their own priorities and plan to inform the health authority of their local perspective. Their work should also take account of policies and priorities conveyed to them from the health authority. In turn the locality group should expect its voice to be heard and acted upon unless, working in partnership with the health authority, it can be persuaded otherwise.

The need for equity

Equity of access according to clinical need is a fundamental, inviolate principle of the NHS. The National Association of Commissioning GPs has adopted the following definition for equity:

> *Equity is the appropriate use of resources within a given population, based upon individual clinical need and agreed criteria of priorities that apply throughout that population.*

It is a more sophisticated principle than at first meets the eye. The most appropriate population will vary for different services. Thus a GP will seek to use his or her time appropriately within a consulting session for the group of patients with appointments for that session. At the same time the preventive services of the practice will be organized to focus on the larger population of the entire practice.

Secondary care requires equity within a larger population again, because the provision of those particular services is for a larger population. Finally, tertiary services involve yet larger populations and here the importance of the principle of equity according to clinical need becomes most apparent.

GP commissioning

Report 6.1: Blackpool Wyre and Fylde GP advisory group

This group was set up by local GPs with support from the LMC and health authority. Nine members represent all GPs within nine localities with a total of 340 000 patients. The nine group members receive sessional payments from the health authority and there is a written agreement defining the relationship between the group and the health authority.

This group demonstrates the effectiveness of GP commissioning. For example, GP concern about local psychiatric services prompted the group to undertake its own enquiries with local specialist colleagues. Subsequent joint work with the health authority resulted in a sum of £700 000 being earmarked for establishing four locality mental health care teams, together with a psychogeriatric service and an enhanced child and adolescent psychiatric service. Major improvements were made in the psychiatric service for all practices and all patients, in a highly efficient, cost-effective manner, in response to GP concern.

Report 6.2: East Dorset commissioning group

Fifty two practices, serving a population of 332 000 patients, are grouped into six localities. Each locality is represented by at least one person in a central core group and there is also a part-time manager who is a local GP. In 1995 funding for the group, from the health authority, was a total of £62 000. This is a striking example of the administrative economies of commissioning compared to fundholding, where that sum would have been spent on the management allowances of two practices alone.

The group has brought about the introduction of open access to ultrasound; the introduction of community-based dermatology services with significant reduction in waiting times; the introduction of 'one stop' neurology clinics leading to reduced waiting times and improved patient convenience; the development of glaucoma screening within primary care in conjunction with the local optical committee; and the development of a community-based audiology service.

Report 6.3: Northamptonshire GP core group

Since 1990 the Northampton Core Group has at all times contained fund-holders and non-fundholders working together. Its strategy throughout has had two elements:

1 working with the statutory authorities concerning commissioning and purchasing

2 working with specialist colleagues to make the best use of existing resources.

While both are successful it is the second which is of particular interest here. Through its specialty liaison groups the core group works with specialists from different disciplines to agree how to make the best use of the resources already available for that discipline, rather than to consider what could be done with additional ones. This simple concept has produced imaginative trade-offs. For example, by negotiating direct access, same day ultrasonography for patients bleeding in the first trimester of pregnancy the service for them has been greatly improved while the number admitted has been reduced by over 50%, producing a net financial saving.

Again, direct, vetted access to the tonsillectomy operating list was introduced in 1992. A specialist receives the completed referral according to an agreed protocol and redirects any to the outpatient clinic about which there is uncertainty. In the first two years this amounted to only 6% of referrals, and over 600 outpatient appointments were released for other patients in greater need of specialist opinion. Overall waiting times were reduced, money saved and many patients saved unnecessary trips to outpatients.

Such co-operation demonstrates how improving services need have nothing to do with 'purchasing' at all. There is a considerable opportunity for health authorities to encourage GPs to work in a co-ordinated manner with their specialist colleagues.

Report 6.4: Nottingham non-fundholders group

This group has 200 GPs caring for nearly 400 000 patients. It is a constituency system of 13 areas, each of which has its own representative on the working group. Representatives on the group are paid on a sessional basis by the health authority. This substantial organization still only cost £66 000 during 1995, or approximately the management allowance for two fundholding practices.

The point to emphasize in this example is the structural work which Nottingham has developed. Its proposed model for total commissioning involving all the GPs in Nottingham was unfortunately rejected by the NHS Executive because it did not fit in with their fundholding strategy, but it is difficult to see any rational explanation why such initiatives should not be enthusiastically supported. Here is a group which has already facilitated an £8.3 million capital investment project to improve ENT, ophthalmology and orthopaedic services. It has established community and practice-based physiotherapy services available to all practices, it has reduced waiting times for first outpatient appointments by as much as 25%, and it has encouraged the appointment of new consultants within specialties where GPs have perceived a particular need. The Nottingham approach to total commissioning has much to commend it within the context of an evolving, primary care-led NHS.

There are many other examples which could be taken from GP commissioning, but the intention here is to demonstrate both the potential and the reality of the approach and the above examples will suffice for that purpose.

How to set up a GP commissioning group

GP commissioning groups are best established by GPs themselves, rather than by the health authority, in order to foster ownership and authority. It is also preferable to do this in conjunction with the LMC, and to start with a meeting to which all GPs are invited, with invitations for representation from the health authority and major providers of secondary care as well. It may also be considered helpful to invite someone from outside the area who has experience of working within a GP commissioning group.

The purpose of the first meeting is to establish if there is a local desire for a representative relationship between the body of GPs and the health authority, regardless of whether they are fundholders or not. If there is then the meeting should establish a working group to get things off the ground. Pragmatism is essential and it is more important at this stage to form the group from enthusiasts than it is to be too concerned with an elected body. That will come later.

The meeting should then agree the preliminary work of the group; areas of responsibility, executive structure, membership structure, requirements for administrative support, and methods of communicating with the practices involved. It is here that the health authority can reasonably be expected to be supportive in terms of finance and administrative facilities.

It is important to establish and maintain momentum. The working group should meet reasonably quickly to address the following issues:

- to establish the aims and objectives of the GP commissioning group

- to agree terminology. To avoid confusion with other agencies who also commission the single word 'commissioning' should be reserved for the collective activity, whether at practice, locality or district level. A suggestion that works in practice is to refer to the overall exercise as commissioning, the GP component as GP commissioning, and the representative group as the (GP) core group

- how to establish a democratic structure that is truly representative. This will commonly be upon a locality basis with elected representatives to a core group

- develop a communications network with appropriate representatives within provider units, the health authority, social services and the community health council, and a proposal for how to communicate with the GP practices themselves

- membership. While the GP commissioning group may initially be made up of GPs alone there is the potential to involve other disciplines and representative groups, perhaps at a locality level

- accountability. The GP core group will be accountable for the opinion it provides to the health authority, but the authority will remain accountable for the budget.

Once the working group has considered these matters it should call another open meeting to allow its conclusions to be discussed. At that stage the mood of all the practices should be assessed, both within the meeting and perhaps by an additional short postal survey. If the response is favourable the GP commissioning group can be formally established and begin its work.

There is a wealth of experience available concerning the work of GP commissioning groups including examples of the crucial, written agreements between groups and their health authorities. The dissemination of that information is a great value of the National Association of Commissioning GPs.

Possible difficulties and disadvantages to look out for

Lack of support from the health authority

The hands of the health authority are tied until the government chooses to release them, though some authorities have been more adventurous than others in their support for GP commissioning. Even then GPs need to ensure that there is a formal working relationship agreed on paper. Very few health authorities so far have appreciated the change required in themselves if they are to work in effective partnership with GPs to develop a primary care-led NHS.

Lack of support from GPs

The considerable advantages of commissioning come to nothing if the participating GPs fail to work within agreed boundaries. At its simplest this requires electing others to represent them and then going along with decisions agreed on their behalf. Commissioning will fail, or at least function sub-optimally, if practices say they will take part but then ignore decisions made collectively by the representative group.

Sensitivity v equity

The greater the sensitivity to the needs of small populations the greater the threat to equity. That is a central dilemma of the NHS internal market and a key criticism of budgets being held at the level of individual practices. The goal of equity within populations of an appropriate size for a given service has been described on page 70.

Information

Commissioning requires information and as discussed earlier there is a pressing need to develop appropriate systems for its collection, collation and dissemination. Again, first and foremost, this requires a political will to do so and for the resources to be made available to support computer development in all practices.

Administrative support

It is remarkable how after five years of GP commissioning there remains no official way to support these groups. While many are resourced by their health authorities, this is discretionary. The resources need to be made available to support the administration of all approaches to involving GPs in developing the NHS.

Payment

GP commissioning is cheap but it is not free. The opportunity costs for GPs involved in commissioning require recompense. This is a different, though related, issue to supporting the administrative infrastructure of the groups.

The need for sophistication

Commissioning is less bureaucratic than fundholding but it is more sophisticated. As such it requires an appropriate infrastructure. Unless those involved realize this its full potential is unlikely to be achieved. The idea that it simply involves a group of non-fundholding GPs offering reactive advice to an all-knowing health authority misses the point by a long way.

The benefits of virement

One of the outstanding advantages of fundholding to date has been to demonstrate the value of viring money from one section of the budget to another. The formation of the health authorities makes that feasible for GP commissioning groups and health authorities working together, if there is a political will to do so. At the same time commissioning GPs should be aware of the potential danger of virement that will shortly threaten fundholding. Virement is fine when there is excess money in the overall budget. However negative equity in the prescribing fund may, out of necessity, soon start to draw money away from that for secondary care, and increasing hospital costs may in turn draw money away from primary care.

Conclusion

This chapter began by identifying four criteria for assessing any approach to GP involvement in developing the NHS. GP commissioning meets all four of those criteria. It is relatively cheap to operate, it has significant advantages when compared to other approaches, and it works. All GPs, fundholders and non-fundholders should feel able to contribute to this approach and work together to improve their local health service.

7

Maintaining quality – the role of audit and education

Ralph Burton

The term 'primary care-led health service' has crept up on us over the last year or two. Like all new terms it seems to have various meanings, some of which are explored in this book. The author would have preferred the term 'community-led health service' as it is clear to him that the terms 'primary' and 'secondary' are rapidly losing their meaning. His task is to examine how audit and education can support this process of change (whatever we call it) and this will depend upon which definition the reader is prepared to accept. For the purposes of this chapter it is assumed that it implies both a shift to the community of much of the work currently undertaken by hospitals and also a responsibility put upon general practice to purchase or commission all that activity which it does not undertake. It therefore includes both provision and purchasing. These two activities are clearly linked but must not be confused, especially when it comes to allocation of resources. The maintenance of quality in health care will thus become a major pre-occupation of general practice both for the work it undertakes and that it gets others to do on its behalf.

Audit or education?

Audit and education are two worthy activities which are used to maintain quality in a professional environment. In the UK education is well established in general practice, with its network of postgraduate centres, advisers and tutors. What was an entirely voluntary system now has an air of compulsion since its linkage to payments in the New Contract introduced in 1990. Recently the traditional providers of education have been joined by a number of other contenders for the privilege of giving GPs their education. These include the family health services authorities (now health authorities), special interest groups, providers of all sorts and the pharmaceutical industry. These 'new kids on the block' of postgraduate education usually have special agendas of their own which they are anxious to have GPs operate. No one can deny that the quantity of education available is adequate; whether this is true of the quality is another matter.

Compared with education, audit is a relative newcomer and has a completely different structure via the medical audit advisory groups (MAAGs) and now, more correctly, the clinical audit advisory groups. These are meant to be independent of their parent FHSAs but rarely are. As education is now compulsory (or you lose money) and audit is not (it is encouraged but is not yet mandatory), they may be viewed as competitors for available time and it is not surprising that education is usually the winner. Despite being widely promoted as a desirable activity by bodies in the UK such as the Royal Colleges of General Practitioners, for many GPs audit remains an activity that is occasionally thought about but rarely done. There are of course many honourable exceptions.

If audit is to fulfil its undoubted potential it will have to enter the mainstream of activity and be seen, together with education, as an essential tool in the delivery of good quality health care. We need to consider what sort of health service we are talking about and to ensure that we have the right structures in place for audit and education to provide adequate support.

What will primary care consist of?

As intimated, the distinctions that exist between primary and secondary care, for a long time rather fuzzy, are now almost totally defunct. What we are referring to is the setting in which most health care will be given, and increasingly this is the community. Within this setting, which will usually be based upon general practice, care will be provided by a mixture of specialists and generalists working together in a number of disciplines. We thus need to know what it is we expect to do within and outwith general practice. Some of this workload shift has already occurred and in certain areas (such as care in the community) it has been accompanied by a resource shift. However, quite often the process has been more *ad hoc*, often not accompanied by any identified resource, and often without adequate agreement. A recent survey has identified some of this activity, which falls into certain categories:

- delegation or subcontracting

- shared care

- pre-referral investigation and pre- and post-operative care

- GP 'sweeper function'.

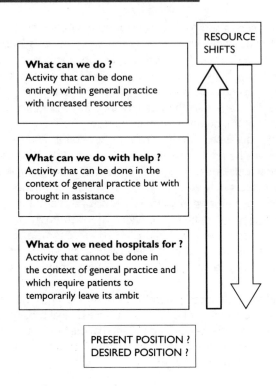

Figure 7.1   Achieving a balance.

These terms are self-explanatory except perhaps for 'sweeper function' which means the activity that a GP picks up unexpectedly as a result of some deficiency in the care system. Clearly such a transfer of work has implications for both resource and education. In addition to not having the means to carry out a task the GP may also not have the knowledge or skills. In addition to achieving a balance within the various aspects of the hospital system, a balance also has to be found between hospital care and general practice (Figure 7.1).

What can general practitioners do?

There are activities which can be performed entirely within general practice by the GP and the primary health care team but which were formerly perceived as the domain of hospital-based care. Exactly where the line is drawn has depended somewhat on the energies and skills of the primary health care team. Referrals to hospitals have varied from the 'please see and treat' variety to patients having been fully investigated, with a specific request for further management. In general, all examinations and investigations necessary to allow a specialist to make a judgement on a single consultation, will have been undertaken by general practice. The general practitioner and the team may also have (or acquire) an extended range of investigation skills such as endoscopy or ultrasonography, or an extended range of treatments such as minor surgery. General practice is usually capable of undertaking all follow-ups after specialist care, sometimes with the help of protocols.

What can general practitioners do with help?

There are also activities which are normally beyond the resources of general practice but which can be achieved with outside assistance. In many practices this will now include the majority of specialist consultations for decisions on further management, best achieved by a tripartite consultation between the patient, the specialist and the GP. The specialist is often able to carry out further tests or treatments within the general practice setting. Expanded general practice teams often include professionals who were formerly entirely hospital-based or from non-health disciplines such as social services or the local authorities. This in turn has facilitated learning, often achieved heuristically, and the development of protocols to enable resources to be more appropriately used.

What do we want hospitals for?

Hospitals are needed for activities which cannot currently be carried out within the context of general practice and which require the patient to be in a different health environment (not necessarily a 'hospital' as we currently know it). This includes the need for equipment or continuous monitoring which cannot be provided in the practice or in the home, or a level of supervision and nursing skills which cannot be provided in the patient's home or nursing home bed. Hospitals are extremely expensive environments and their use should be restricted to patients who have an absolute need for their services. Without this saving no resource shift will be possible.

A practical example of this approach; linked to contracting

By way of example a specific condition (prostatism) is shown as a contracting exercise (Figure 7.2). In this example it could be argued that the total cost of the episode of care is more or less equally divided between general practice and the hospital, although currently, usually 100% will go to the hospital-based provider, no matter how much is done in general practice. The arrows A, B and C demonstrate the types of contract that a purchaser could set, depending on the workload shift. Clearly contracts at B or C will have implications on quality, as well as resource, and thus on the provision of education and audit.

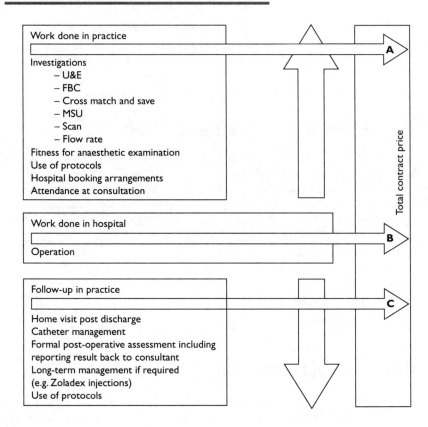

Figure 7.2 Contracting for change; example – prostatism.

Audit

One simple definition of audit is that it is the process of systematically looking at one's work with the aim of doing it better. This simple objective has a number of prerequisites (Figure 7.3). However, unless there is a willingness to change, and to demonstrate such change, audit can become merely an accounting procedure and is best described as quality control. This applies to most data collected from general practices, such as those used to monitor target payments. This is not audit but can become so when it induces change. This may occur from nothing more high minded than the wish to reach a target payment but can be matched to any number of other standards available to general practice.

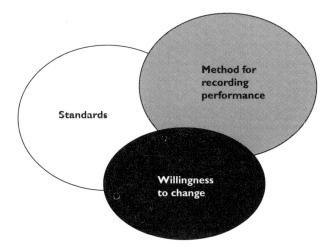

Figure 7.3 The prerequisites for audit.

Education

Education would seem to have much the same aim as audit: to systematically increase or at least modify the amount we know with the aim of improving performance. Education and audit now seem to be opposite sides of the same coin and are no longer competitors for time and resource. All audit is educational but, as yet, not all education is audit (although it could be argued that it should be, for what use is it in this context unless it makes a demonstrable difference to performance?). If the link is made between audit and education then a new audit–education cycle emerges (Figure 7.4).

Figure 7.4 shows that if a GP agrees to give an educator (whoever that may be) audit data together with their defined standards, it should be possible to devise an educational programme which addresses their identified needs. This should allow them to perform better and any improvement can be demonstrated by re-audit. Thus audit should be capable of defining what it is they need to know and also be able to measure the value of the educational process.

Audit directed education

It seems logical that audit and education be linked together to make a common activity which is appropriate, effective and economical with the use of time. The principles behind this are:

- the aims of education and audit are fundamentally the same and should be viewed as varying perspectives of the same activity

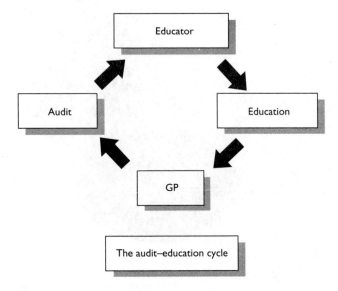

Figure 7.4   The audit–education cycle.

- auditing performance against agreed standards should tell educationalists what individuals need to know and re-audit will give information about the effectiveness of the delivery of that education.

Attempts are being made to put these principles into practice by getting those charged with promoting audit to work alongside those similarly charged with education in producing common programmes. Inevitably both activities are being looked at by health service managers as possible ways by which their agendas may be fulfilled and they are not likely to remain funded as free floating entities. Efforts will have to be made to ensure that the activities that doctors wish to carry out are congruent with the aims and aspirations of those who hold the purse strings. If we can include as many themes as possible within a single programme we may help GPs to feel a little less under siege from the high levels of demand. Some of the current and future influences are:

- Health of the Nation
- care in the community
- Patient's Charter
- new contract
- summative assessment
- reaccreditation
- educational initiatives such as mentoring and portfolio learning

- service initiatives such as extended and total fundholding

- evidenced-based medicine.

Integrated learning

Bringing the strands together is a vital task if we are to make maximum use of professional time, avoid duplication and still ensure that we develop a high quality service. This should be the true aim behind a primary care-led health service and standards will need to be vigorously defended. The author has worked within a practical programme that recognized all these entities; audit, education and service provision, and tried to integrate them in a common activity for a year-on-year programme. The content of such a programme needs to be negotiated with as many stakeholders as possible, most importantly the GPs and the rest of the primary health care team, and with the health authorities.

The aim of the programme was to make a system so specific that it could be operated at practice level, or even with each individual GP, but initially it had to be started at a district level. To decide what the priorities should be information which was already available was used, which included:

- prescribing data

- morbidity data

- health promotion data

- audit reports to support special payments.

As long as these data were linked to standards, not averages, and the practices were willing to change when necessary, audit could be obtained without struggling to establish new layers of data collection. Inevitably, the targets set out in the Health of the Nation were a priority so it was decided to find out which elements were most important to a particular district and to use this as the basis of the three way negotiation. Figure 7.5 shows the national, regional and district variance from the Health of the Nation targets.

This demonstrated that a programme concentrating on under-aged pregnancy, suicide and cervical cancer was unlikely to have as much influence as one taking cardiovascular risk factors and stroke as its main theme. In the end four areas were agreed and formed the basis of the programme. To promote the programme in the practices and to encourage individual audit, practices were able to call upon the services of an educational mentor who was available to visit them. Figure 7.6 shows what the programme eventually looked like. The health authority agreed to sponsor the programme as its principle route to achieving its requirement under the Health of the Nation agenda.

Well established principles of adult learning need to be applied if education is to be successful. It must be seen to be relevant to perceived need and should be

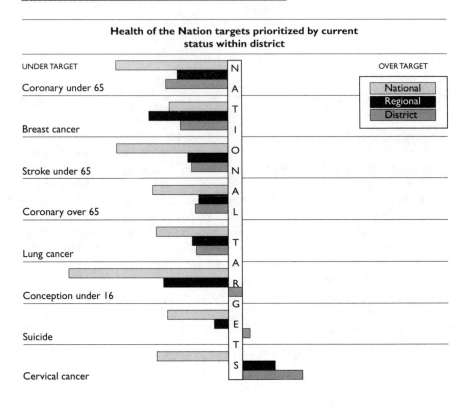

Figure 7.5 National, regional and district variance from Health of the Nation targets.

offered in ways which maximize learning opportunity. In general practice, this increasingly means going to the practice and involving the whole of the multidisciplinary team. Learners need to feel that they are engaged in a shared exercise and are not being preached to; this requires acknowledgement of their previous life experience and using that as a knowledge base. Many blocks develop to the reception and integration of new learning and a skilled mentor can help to identify and overcome these. The role of a mentor will thus include:

- identifying gaps in knowledge and an awareness of available resources
- being skilled in adult education concepts and their application to general practice
- having sufficient understanding of audit to allow its development as a tool for deciding educational need and judging educational outcome
- identifying the preferred learning styles of individuals and teams
- addressing blocks to learning.

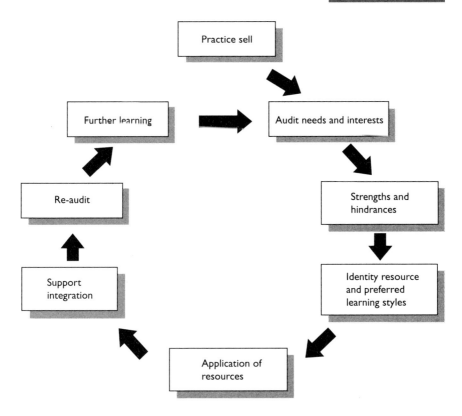

Figure 7.6   The project process/work with the practice.

Conclusion

A primary care-led health service is a term which reflects and emphasizes the many changes that have occurred in the purchasing and provision of medical services in the UK over the last half a decade. The pace of change has almost overwhelmed us and is multifactorial but essentially defines a shift of care from an institutional setting to the community. Because of the established structure most of this is going to be centred on general practice although by no means will all of it be provided by general practitioners. General practitioners will however have a key role in the provision of services that they have traditionally seen as the province of others, and in the purchasing of those services that they do not themselves provide. If standards are to be preserved, and in many instances improved, the process will need to be underwritten by a robust system of audit and education. This chapter has tried to show that these are complementary activities which can be usefully combined in support of service provision. This would be best achieved by new partnerships between those responsible for audit, those with educational briefs and service providers together with health service purchasers of all types. No one group alone is likely to make much impact but working together it should be possible not only to maintain quality but to deliver improvements. As Professor Marshall Marinker recently said, 'Donabedian's original trilogy of structure, process and outcome has now been stood on its head'. We now need to ask first what it is we wish to achieve and follow this by looking at the processes most likely to produce those desired outcomes and then finally defining the structure in which this can be best achieved. If we have learnt anything, then it is that there is nothing permanent about structure which cannot be blown away as easily as sand in the wind.

8

Hospital – a primary, secondary care interface

Christina Victor

It is estimated that five million people in Great Britain are admitted as in-patients to acute hospitals each year, a third as emergencies. For most people admission to hospital represents a crisis, and is a highly significant event in their lives. Patients worry about how they will manage to take care of themselves and their home, about the prospects for their future health and whether they will be able to lead a 'normal life' once they are discharged back home. Therefore while a primary care-led service covers many aspects of care, it is often this interface with the secondary care services that colours most people's perception of the ability of a health service to cope. Almost since the inception of the NHS, problems have been experienced when trans-ferring responsibility for patients between the primary and secondary care sectors. There are three main areas of concern:

1   problems of communication between hospital and community

2   the experiences of 'vulnerable' groups as exemplified by the elderly

3   delayed discharge.

Communication between hospital and community

Patients rarely understand the different roles and responsibilities of the primary and secondary health care sectors. Furthermore it is highly unlikely that they fully com-prehend the remit of the social care agencies. For many patients and carers, admission to hospital represents, in their eyes, a continuation of their care and not as an event which involves responsibility for their care moving between different types of doctors. However, the organization of the NHS since its inception has distinguished between the primary and secondary sectors and communication between them remains problematic. The separation of responsibility for the provision of 'social' care to the local authorities adds another layer of complexity which has to be overcome when arranging for the care of patients, especially those with complex needs such as elderly people.

Communication between doctors working in primary and secondary care sectors is largely effected via referral and discharge letters. This apparently simple and uncomplicated arrangement has spawned a vast research literature but one which has concentrated upon communication on discharge; communication between doctors when patients are admitted has been subject to much less research.

Entering hospital

Admissions may be planned in advance or as a result of an emergency. The route of admission taken by a patient will strongly influence the knowledge a general practitioner has of this event. If an admission is organized as a result of an intervention by the general practitioner then clearly they are aware that the event has taken place. However, for emergency and, to a lesser extent, for admissions planned well in advance the general practitioner may be unaware or uncertain that the event has taken place. A study in inner London reported that amongst house staff surveyed only about a third, 34%, routinely contacted the general practitioner when an older person was admitted. This was echoed by a GP surveyed as part of this study: 'It is unacceptable that there is no longer a routine system to notify the primary care team that a patient has been admitted'.[1]

Leaving hospital

The established practice at discharge is for a short discharge summary to be sent by the hospital to the patient's GP, followed by a longer, hopefully more informative discharge letter. This arrangement was reported as operating in the majority (87%) of geriatric medical units in a recent survey and this is indicative of the widespread and routine nature of this system. Two areas have dominated the discharge letter debate: what information should be included and how can delays in communication between primary and secondary care be reduced? Most studies have highlighted the dissatisfaction of general practitioners with the information included in discharge letters which in a minority of cases affected their management of the case. Victor et al.[1] report that in their study only 41% of GPs reported that discharge notification from the study hospitals for older people was good or very good. The main issues around the contents of the discharge letter have been the failure of the communication to contain sufficient details of the diagnosis, the outcome of investigations/tests undertaken in hospital and drug regimens, especially where drugs had been stopped or started in hospital. A comment made by a practitioner illustrates these issues: 'Often results of assessments made in hospital are not communicated to GPs. No recommendations for management after assessment is also a problem'.

General practitioners were disturbed by the small supply of drugs often prescribed by hospitals at discharge and the failure of hospitals to indicate to patients that they need to contact their GP for continuation of medication.

For older patients there have been attempts to improve the quality of discharge information by the development of check lists and standardized letters. In theory at least it should be possible for primary and secondary care staff to agree on locally specific standard discharge letters. However, this remains a challenge which is largely unanswered. The development of fundholding may become the mechanism by which hospital–primary care information transfer can be improved at both admission and discharge from hospital.

Another serious issue is the delay which can occur in communication between hospital and primary care. A distinction must be drawn here between the short discharge letter and the more detailed discharge summary. Penney[2] reported that 80% of discharge letters between hospital and primary care arrived within one week, although in this case they were delivered in person by the patient. However, when considering discharge summaries Penney reported that 11% arrived within one week and just over a third, 39%, within 14 days; a quarter never arrived. Similarly Black[3] found that a discharge summary could take between one day and four months to arrive. In that study the main reason for the delay appeared to be lack of secretarial and administrative support in the hospital. Victor et al.[4] have also drawn attention to the lack of administrative support for the discharge process, of which preparation and distribution of discharge letters and summaries is one aspect. Clearly increased use of new technology such as fax machines and hospital–primary care computer links could expedite the process of information transfer. The development of contracting and purchasing should prove to be a means by which levels of communication across the interface are improved. Fundholding and the development of GP collectives may also prove effective mechanisms for improving the transfer of information between different segments of the health care system.

Involving community and social services

It is to nursing staff that much of the responsibility for co-ordinating discharge and linking with the social care agencies falls. However discharge-related data are often missing from nursing notes because of their concentration on inpatient care and treatment. It is not simply with the GP that the hospital needs to communicate. Rather they need to be in touch with nursing and other health service staff and the social care agencies. There are the same inadequacies and shortcomings of the system: little warning of a patient's impending discharge from hospital, poor quality of information supplied and the late arrival of discharge letters. Furthermore hospital-based staff are not always fully aware of the availability and role of community-based health services or the social care agencies. As a doctor reported: 'I think the hospital staff have unrealistic expectations of what community care can be provided'.

Again there is no obvious formal mechanism for feedback between hospital and community-based nursing staff which would enable the two care sectors to become more aware of what each can realistically provide. The same applies to social services. Marks[5] comments that a study conducted by Brent Social Services highlighted the lack of formal procedures between hospitals and social service departments: no mechanisms for notification when social service clients were admitted, short notice of discharge and the lack of a formal feedback mechanism.

Who should be responsible for organizing and facilitating discharge? Victor et al.[4] point to the ambiguities and informality of many current arrangements. In their study doctors talked to community medical staff, nurses talked to nurses and it was unclear whose responsibility it was to liaise with non-health services. As one nurse stated: 'I personally object to having to arrange social services for the patients'.

One mechanism suggested as a means of improving communication between the different stakeholders involved in discharge has been via the creation of specialist discharge liaison posts. However, there has been a lack of clarity about the precise role of liaison staff. Is it to promote the mutual education of the hospital and community staff, is it to determine patients who 'need' discharge planning or is it to arrange the actual discharge? This lack of certainty about their function has resulted in an ambiguity about their usefulness. Victor et al.[1] have drawn attention to the difficulties potentially experienced by liaison staff when they have no control over resources and no management 'clout' to make things happen. Such posts could easily be typified as having responsibility without power.

Discharge and older people

Almost since the inception of the NHS concern has been expressed by a variety of different agencies about the post-hospital discharge problems experienced by older people. Despite the varying 'professional' origins of the researchers/projects (e.g. doctors, GPs, nurses and social workers) research in this field has consistently identified six recurrent problems.[5] Each of these are briefly considered.

Home circumstances not discussed

Older people who are in contact with the accident and emergency service or who are treated as inpatients on acute medical wards are not routinely asked about their home circumstances. Nor does it appear that they are systematically asked as to how they will cope at home after they have been discharged. Between one-half and one-third of older people in a variety of studies could not recall hospital staff asking them how they would manage at home. It is unclear as to whether there has been a radical change in this area since the introduction of community care in 1993.

Little information given

Older people do not recall being given information about their diagnosis, medication, potential side effects of drugs and any 'appropriate' lifestyle changes which they should make as a result of their condition.

Patients and carers not involved in discharge planning

The contribution carers make to the care of older people and other dependent groups in the community is now documented and is supposed to be central under the new community care arrangements. However, they remain largely uninvolved in the discharge planning process. As one respondent stated: 'You tell them (the relatives) the date of discharge … If they are unhappy about the discharge you ask them to make an appointment to see the consultant'.

Hospital doctors' lack of knowledge of discharge policies

With the implementation of the Community Care Act there is a much greater emphasis upon locally agreed policies and joint working. However it is apparent many junior doctors are unaware of the policies for organizing discharge from hospital. Failure to provide sufficient notice of an impending discharge is a strong theme which has featured in virtually every study conducted over the last three decades. Approximately one-third of patients over 65 were given 24 hours or less notice of their impending discharge. Bowling and Betts[6] reported that a quarter of their sample were given no notice of discharge. Even where a discharge has been well planned changes in hospital circumstances may result in the plans being changed at the last moment. Victor et al.[1] report that one older person in their study was discharged in a rush. The ward sister reported that: 'she (the patient) was discharged very quickly in the end. There was a bed rush on … She was supposed to be going on a home visit which ended up being she could stay at home … her son came back and collected her stuff …'.

Community services do not commence on time

Finally, problems with transport and the failure of community services to commence when people arrive back home has been an enduring feature of research studies. One result of this failure to provide adequate after-care has been that a significant minority of older people feel that they have been discharged home too early.

Delayed discharge

The recent Audit Commission Report[7] draws attention to the need to use scarce acute inpatient beds 'appropriately'. This report represents the most recent manifestation of an important part of the hospital discharge literature which is concerned with 'blocked' beds or delayed discharge. This again is a long-standing and widespread problem. In the 1970s the majority of (90 out of 94) area health authorities surveyed reported that they had a problem with 'blocked' acute beds. A large body of research has sought to enumerate the size of the problem (using increasingly sophisticated methods such as the Oxford Bed Study Instrument) and its causes. The focus of research has moved away from a narrow concentration upon the person perceived as occupying a 'blocked' bed to an analysis concerned with overall management of acute care and its role and functions. Poor and haphazard discharge planning is a contributory factor to the problem, which has significant costs for both the providers, and often forgotten, consumers of care.

Another aspect of the hospital discharge issue relating to the 'blocking' of acute beds is concerned with the use of acute beds by people awaiting placement in long-term care. In inner London it has been reported that 13% of acute beds were being used inappropriately.[1] Provision of a 'homefinder service' dedicated to locating appropriate, private sector long-term care has been proposed as one way of reducing inappropriate acute hospital bed use. However, again the evidence to support the development of such services is largely descriptive. It is unclear as to whether the implementation of the Community Care Act has reduced this problem or exacerbated it by the lengthy nature of the assessment process.

Responding to the identified problems: the development of a hospital discharge policy

The long history of problems of discharge from acute medical care back to the primary care and social care sectors is obvious. The consistency and similarity of the problems identified is striking given the extensive degree of variation exhibited in the research designs employed in these studies. What solutions have been suggested for these well rehearsed problems? Marks[5] notes that solutions have been sought in the successive re-organizations of the NHS which have tried to provide clear lines of managerial responsibility between the primary, secondary and social care sectors and to improve the co-ordination of care between agencies. However such bureaucratic re-organizations have achieved only limited success.

Central guidance on hospital discharge was issued in 1989. The Department of Health circular HC(89)5 and accompanying booklet *Discharge of Patients from Hospital* sought to improve discharge planning for patients of all ages by stressing the need to ensure that proper arrangements for the return home and any required after-care should be organized before discharge. The main recommendations of this circular are summarized in Box 8.1 and revolve around early planning of discharge, written policies, good communication and the centrality of patients and carers in the process.

Marks[5] has considered the limitations of the circular and notes that it concentrates upon professional accountability and does not confer any 'rights' in determining discharge upon either patients or their carers. She also observes that the circular remains very vague about certain aspects of discharge, especially the point of responsibility transfer between hospital and community.

Box 8.1   Key points of health circular HC(89)5.

- Establishing discussion procedures

  - procedures to be agreed with all involved in their implementation

  - all wards and departments to agree discharge procedures which should be issued to all concerned

  - procedures to be monitored by DHA in association with local authorities

  - RHAs to be informed of action taken

- Creating effective arrangements

  - doctors responsible for patient to agree discharge

  - doctors to have agreed and managers to be satisfied that arrangements for home care are comprehensive

  - one member of staff to hold responsibility for seeing that all necessary action has been taken prior to discharge

  - information from patients to be incorporated into reviews of discharge policies

  - consultants play an important role in the review of procedures along with a range of other professionals

  - procedures to be circulated to GPs, ambulance service, social services, housing departments and any relevant voluntary bodies

---

The implementation of the community care reforms in April 1993 changed the policy context fundamentally by giving the local authority the lead responsibility for social care. Of the eight key tasks for local authorities implementing the community care reforms, one is concerned directly with arrangements for hospital discharge and two are indirectly related to this (assessment of individuals for continuing care and clarifying arrangements for continuing care). Clearly systems for the assessment of needs of individuals (for long-term or care at home) must work within a framework of agreements for hospital discharge. However there is a tension between the macro health perspective concerned with optimal use of hospital resources and micro level social service perspectives concerned with individual-based assessment and choice.

The ideas enshrined in the 1989 circular have been further developed in the *Hospital Discharge Workbook*[8] developed by the Department of Health and Social Services inspectorate. The workbook contains illustrations of good practice and looks at the various stages which make up 'the discharge process', and attempts to view each stage from the perspectives of the main stakeholders. It clearly has a number of applications, most of which are again concerned with the identification of managerial responsibilities and audit.

Box 8.2 Elements of 'good' hospital discharge as defined by patients and carers

- Heating should be turned on in the house on morning of discharge.
- Fresh staple goods should be in the house.
- One meal should be ready for the person returning home.
- Home carer should be waiting if there are no relatives/friends.
- 24–48 hours' notice should be given of discharge.
- Discharge timing should be specific (e.g. a.m. or p.m.).
- Services in place on day of discharge.
- Services post-discharge should be provided seven days a week.
- GP should be on call on day of discharge.
- Nurses should be available to 'tuck down' at night.
- Procedures need to be established to give keys to carers before discharge.
- It should be ensured that there is a carer available who will accept responsibility and who is physically able.
- A single member of hospital staff should have responsibility for arranging this.

Adapted from Barnes and Cormie[9]

Putting the needs of carers and patients at the centre of service planning and development is a rhetoric which is often expressed. However it is rarer for the experiences of users and carers to be taken as the 'core' of service development. Barnes and Cormie[9] report the results of a study undertaken with older people discharged from hospital in Scotland. Drawing on their own experiences the users highlighted the short notice of discharge, waiting for transport and failure to provide services as promised. Box 8.2 summarizes the issues raised by this user group.

Conclusions

Length of stay, once admitted to hospital, has been decreasing for older people (and indeed other age groups). A high admission rate combined with a short and decreasing length of stay may be indicative of an 'efficient' use of a scarce resource such as acute hospital beds. However, such aggressive modes of service delivery may result in problems in planning discharge of people and in developing appropriate links with the community services which they may require once they are back home.

Another suggested side-effect of poor discharge planning and after-care is re-admission to hospital. Indeed it has been suggested that readmission rates may be a surrogate indicator of the 'quality' of discharge planning received by patients. There is obviously no 'simple' correlation between readmission and the quality of the initial treatment and subsequent discharge back home. Some readmissions are planned and some readmissions are for another unrelated condition. Clearly these types of readmission do not give any indication of the quality of the initial treatment and discharge. Only unplanned readmissions for the same condition occurring fairly quickly (e.g. within 7–14 days) after the initial discharge may be related to either the quality of care received in hospital or the quality of the care provided in the community. Data from both Scotland[10] and Oxford report the increase in emergency readmission over the last decade whilst Townsend et al.[11] highlight the problems of readmission amongst older people and that these can be reduced by the provision of appropriate after-care. A significant percentage of readmissions could be avoided with appropriate care after discharge. There are failures in the current system and a number of authors suggest potential ways that more targeted 'post-discharge support' could be provided.

There is a wealth of descriptive evidence available about the 'failure' of current procedures for the discharge of older people. Evidence to indicate the best ways of improving the very obvious deficiencies in the current system of discharge is rather sparse. Many descriptive studies have supported the setting up of hospital discharge schemes designed to facilitate early and less problematic discharge. However, evaluation of the effectiveness of such schemes has been limited and the results not very optimistic. Two evaluative studies looked at the effectiveness of specially designed hospital discharge schemes using a randomized controlled trial. In Wales the randomized controlled trial study design was not complied with by the staff providing the service and the data had to be analysed using a case-control method. The study showed that the scheme failed to meet its objectives of achieving earlier discharge. Townsend et al.[12] evaluated a scheme to provide post-discharge support to those aged 75+. Over the 18 month trial period there was a halving of the readmission rate (6.7% in the intervention group and 13.9% in the control group) and the control group spent an average of 25% more days in hospital.

It is too early to comment with any degree of certainty about the way that the implementation of caring for people has influenced the way the interfaces between primary, secondary and social care operate. However in order for the new arrangements to work four issues must be addressed:

1   ensuring that discharge does not take place before assessment has taken place, a care plan agreed and resources put in place

2   procedures for the assessment and care plan development need to be agreed

3   mechanisms for involving users and carers need to be agreed

4   there needs to be an agreed process for transferring care plans from hospital to community.

Many of these issues touch upon the long-standing problems which have been identified in the relationship between the primary, secondary and social care sectors. In evaluation and monitoring the success of the community care reforms we may need to distinguish long-term structural problems from those resultant from the implementation of the Act. However, if the Act is to work good practice, as exemplified by written agreements and joint working, will become mandatory; without it there will be no improvement in the way the health and social agencies work for the effective discharge of people from hospital back to the community.

References

1   Victor CR, Young E, Hudson M et al. (1993) Whose responsibility is it anyway? Hospital admission and discharge of older people in an inner London DHA. Journal of Advanced Nursing. **18**: 1297–1304.

2   Penney T. (1988) Delayed communication between hospitals and general practitioners: where does the problem lie. British Medical Journal. **297**: 28–9.

3   Black D. (1990) How to do justice to discharge … Geriatric Medicine. **29**: 9.

4   Victor CR, Young E, Wallace P. (1991) Older people at the interface, occasional paper No.2. Daniels Press, Cambridge.

5   Marks L. (1994) Seamless care or patchwork quilt: discharging patients from acute hospital care. King's Fund Institute Research Report No.17.

6   Bowling A, Betts G. (1984) Communication on discharge. Nursing Times. **8 April**: 31–3.

7   Audit Commission. (1992) Lying in wait. HMSO, London.

8   DoH. (1994) The Hospital Discharge Workbook. HMSO, London.

9   Barnes M, Cormie J. (1995) On the panel. Health Service Journal. **213**: 30–1.

10   Henderson J, Goldacre MJ, Simmons HM et al. (1989) Use of medical record linkage to study readmission rates. British Medical Journal. **299**: 709–13.

11   Townsend J. (1992) Emergency hospital admissions and readmissions of patients aged 75 years and over and the effects of a community-based discharge scheme. Health Trends. **24**: 136–9.

12   Townsend J, Piper M, Frank AO et al. (1988) Reduction in hospital readmission stay of elderly patients by a community-based hospital discharge scheme: a randomised controlled trial. British Medical Journal. **297**: 544–7.

9

Role of the new health authorities

Siân Griffiths and Jonathan McWilliam

Health authorities with responsibility for primary and secondary care came into being in April 1996. The new structure is the result of the changes announced in October 1993 which merged district health authorities and family health services authorities. These new single health authorities take on responsibility for the regulation and management of primary care services at a local level and integrate purchasing across primary and secondary care. In anticipation of the legislation, many DHAs and FHSAs have already been working much more closely together and have merged their functions and management structures.

The same legislation will also abolish the old regional health authorities, which will become part of the civil service as regional offices of the NHS Executive. These changes are outlined in Figures 9.1 and 9.2.

The changes, when considered together, have far reaching implications for a primary care-led NHS, some of which are explicit and some of which are less obvious. This chapter attempts to describe clearly the changes, firstly for health authorities themselves and secondly for GPs and primary care. The chapter concludes with an assessment of the challenges to be faced.

What do the changes mean for health authorities?

The key implications of changes are:

1 a single health strategy spanning primary and secondary care
2 a uniform approach, spanning primary and secondary care, to:

- disease management

- purchasing services

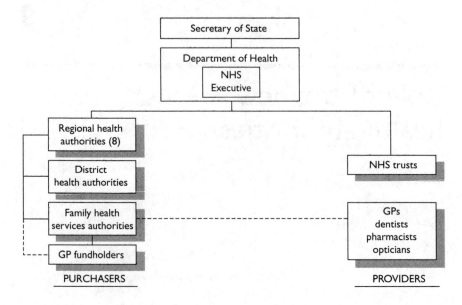

Figure 9.1 Simplified structure of the NHS, pre-April 1996.

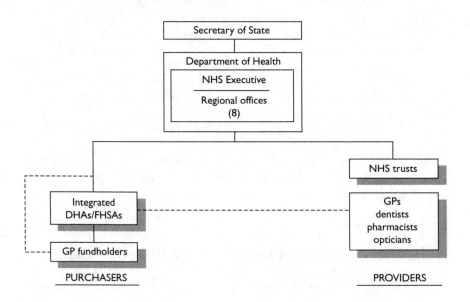

Figure 9.2 Simplified structure of the NHS, post-April 1996.

- quality of care

- finance

- priority setting

3   responding to the public.

A common health strategy

A health strategy is a forward view of how health care services should develop for a given population. In general a health strategy is based on three questions:

1   where are we now?

2   where do we want to be?

3   how are we going to get there?

A single health authority for a given geographical patch will be better positioned to assess the health status and health care needs of the people living within its boundaries, and develop a perspective on the whole spectrum of care, such as:

- health promotion (tobacco advertising)

- disease prevention (health checks)

- treatment (thrombolysis)

- rehabilitation (use of leisure centres)

- care (after-care in the community).

It also makes possible the 'health care programme approach', a means of developing a clinical consensus on how to manage diseases in a consistent way whether in primary, secondary or tertiary care.

Assessment of health care needs

Health authorities are responsible for health as well as for health services within their patch. Understanding how healthy a population is, and what their health care needs may be, is one of their key roles. Epidemiological data from a variety of sources can be put together to form a picture of health care needs. Services for groups such as elderly people or the physically disabled can now be planned using data such as:

- census data

- national survey data e.g. on disabilities

- trends in GP consultations

- trends in GP referrals

- data from district nurses

- care management data from social services

- hospital data

- local information about patients'/the public's views.

These data can help to clarify mis-matches between what is needed and what exists. Information on health needs is the basis of the health strategy which informs the purchasing process. The assessment of health care needs for elderly people should therefore shape the health strategy, which in turn will shape purchasing of services, which has implications for the work of GPs and their teams, for district nurses working for community trusts and for clinicians working in hospitals.

Increasingly efforts are being made to use data to assess the quality of care, the health outcome of interventions and the patients' views (Figure 9.3).

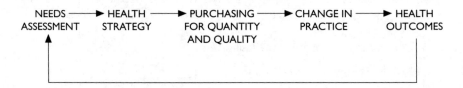

Figure 9.3   Data used to assess the quality of care, the health outcome of interventions and the patients' views.

Disease management

The health care programme approach

The health care programme approach takes a clinical area, e.g. the management of coronary heart disease, and considers what interventions might be carried out across the whole spectrum of health care. For coronary heart disease this might include:

- health promotion/disease prevention

- primary care/community care

- secondary care

- after-care.

Taking this approach assists in viewing patients in a holistic way. It is also useful for balancing the competing demands of different treatments which can be carried out in different settings, e.g. what is the role of primary care versus the role of secondary care in the management of angina? How much money should we invest in health promotion, and how much in invasive surgery? This approach looks across the traditional primary/secondary divide; a process made easier by the creation of new authorities.

The purchasing process

How does a strategy relate to purchasing?

The process of purchasing health care is one of the main tasks of a health authority, increasingly being shared with primary care in a variety of different ways (see chapters five and six). Creating a single health strategy for primary and secondary care will improve the new health authority's ability to purchase integrated services with GPs, from community services and hospital services. This is not however a straightforward matter. For example, at least the following activities need to be co-ordinated:

- negotiating contracts with trusts for volume, price and quality care within hospitals and the community
- working together with GP fundholders to co-ordinate purchasing
- negotiating with all GPs to change/agree ways of working
- negotiating with other organizations, e.g. social services to co-ordinate efforts.

In an ideal world the purchasing process would be based on health care needs assessment translated into purchasing plans and contracts to produce desired outcomes for a defined population. In practice there are, however, many factors apart from needs and resources which influence the health policy process such as political directives, local opinions and geographical factors. At the end of the day the process has much less clarity and decisions have to be made with the best information available within existing resources. It is the health authority's responsibility to achieve the best balance.

Quality – how does it fit in?

A main responsibility for health authorities is to purchase services of high quality. The re-organized NHS gives new opportunities for approaching quality of care in a uniform way across primary and secondary care. The quality of care is monitored against a set of criteria:

- *effectiveness*. The extent to which something achieves what it sets out to achieve, e.g. are new treatments shown to have a therapeutic effect in clinical trials?
- *efficiency*. The extent to which the maximum effect is achieved for a given input or the extent to which an input can be minimized to produce a given effect,

e.g. day surgery is said to be more efficient because the cost of overnight stay in hospital is avoided

- *equity*. The extent to which something is comparably fair, e.g. the different ways in which different socio-economic groups make use of health services may contribute to the widening gap in health status between rich and poor. How can services be modified to reverse this effect?

- *accessibility*. The ease with which individuals or groups can utilize health services, e.g. are rural communities disadvantaged when compared with urban communities because of the greater average distances between their homes and primary health care teams?

- *appropriateness*. To what extent the right intervention is delivered in the right place for the right person, e.g. is methadone an appropriate treatment for drug addiction, and if so, should it be prescribed by GPs or consultants?

- *responsiveness*. The extent to which services are in keeping with the wishes of the public or the wishes of the individual.

It is the task of the health authorities to purchase services which improve quality as measured by the criteria above. This is not easy for several reasons:

- the starting point may be far from the ideal level of quality. This means that improvement may be slow

- quality criteria may conflict and a compromise has to be struck, e.g. vaccination is effective, efficient and appropriate, but periodic 'scares' about the safety of different vaccines can make them unacceptable to the public

- it is short-sighted to see the effects of health care in isolation, e.g. day surgery may be more efficient for hospital services, but more expensive to society as a whole when the extra burden placed on carers is taken into account

- good monitoring and outcome measures are few in number and expensive to carry out

- good quality depends on your point of view. GPs and consultants for example frequently differ in their opinions about good quality care. The reasons for this are complex, but include: the different characteristics of the different populations they treat; their differing philosophies with regard to 'holistic' approaches and 'single-organ' approaches to treatment and their different thresholds for initiating investigation and treatment. A challenge of the new health authorities is to understand and reconcile these differences within a single strategy.

Financial issues

Perhaps the biggest challenge for health authorities in undertaking their work is to balance the financial books. One of the anxieties often expressed about the merging of primary and secondary care is that the demands for specialist care will mean that primary and community care will suffer. One of the health authorities' responsibilities will be to ensure that a proper balance is kept between different parts of the service.

At present, money comes into the new health authorities through two main sources. In simplified terms, one source funds hospital and community trust services and the other funds general practice, NHS dentistry, community pharmacy and some optometry services. These two sources of money are allocated and used in different ways. For example, within non-fundholding primary health care teams, district nurse and health visitor services are negotiated locally with community trusts from one source of funding, while payments for GPs' services and money for practice nursing and practice staff comes from a second funding route. This can act as a barrier to purchasing an integrated service.

Some argue that the current way of funding primary care – via a nationally negotiated contract – needs to be changed and there should be a move towards a single way of funding all health services. This may happen in the future, but at present it is not part of the current organizational changes. The new health authorities will continue to manage the money for GPs in much the same way as the FHSAs would have done, and at the same time, will also be purchasing health care from the acute and community trusts (along with GP fundholders) with money from a different route. The task of the new health authorities is to use these two routes as though they were the same because this is the only way to achieve integrated services.

Priorities and rationing

One of the major differences in perspective between primary care practitioners and policy makers within health authorities is that the former are primarily concerned with the benefit possible for an individual patient whereas the latter are concerned with the greater good for groups of patients. The balance between the needs of individuals and the needs of groups in the population means that at times some patients may not be able to have the required treatment because it is of lower priority within the strategic and purchasing frameworks of a district. The debate about prioritization, or more crudely, rationing, is set to become more open because the three main drivers of demand for health care are likely to increase. These drivers are:

- demographic (the increasing elderly population)
- technical (the increasing availability of advanced scientific interventions and new and expensive drugs)
- public demand (members of the public are becoming increasingly more know-ledgeable and more articulate in their demands from the health care system).

The challenge for new health authorities is to make decisions about priorities which are consistent across primary and secondary care. These decisions should also take into account the advice of the public and professionals from primary, secondary and tertiary care.

Responding to the public

Patient demand and the government's emphasis on consumer involvement in the health service place an additional responsibility on health authorities to ensure that their local public are informed and involved in health care decisions in primary and secondary care. Effective consultation in both sectors is a developing area of work. The real challenge lies in reflecting the public's views on a comprehensive health strategy in a meaningful way.

Formal processes

The creation of new health authorities allows similar formal processes of the DHAs and FHSAs to be amalgamated. These are presented below, for the sake of completeness, as a simple list:

- **complaints** from the public against practitioners, hospitals or purchasers
- monitoring the **Patient's Charter** and the **primary care charter**
- monitoring **prescribing** by GPs and hospitals
- arrangements for **medical audit** in primary and secondary care.

What do the changes mean for GPs and primary care teams?

More say for local GPs

The trend requiring both FHSAs and DHAs to work more closely with local general practitioners is likely to continue and develop. This gives GPs an unprecedented influence over the hospital and community services that are purchased. This development is more likely to bring about a primary care-led NHS than any other. The extent to which health services can be planned from the point of view of primary care is greatly increased.

The influence of GPs will however be strongest where it is best co-ordinated. There are many ways in which GPs can group together to speak with a single voice, including:

- traditional routes such as the Local Medical Committee (LMC) and subgroups of the LMC

- local GPs meeting in small geographical 'localities' based perhaps around issues specific to parts of a city, town or rural area

- local groups of GP fundholders meeting to co-ordinate both their own purchasing and how to influence DHA purchasing

- GPs seconded to work within health authorities, concentrating either on specific issues and/or contracts with specific trusts

- projects to extend GP fundholding.

Stronger primary health care teams

Different methods of funding, and different management structures have frequently created tensions in the primary health care team between, for example, GPs/ practice nurses on the one hand and health visitors/district nurses on the other. The new organization has the potential to work with LMCs and community trusts to reduce these historic tensions and therefore increase the strength of primary health care teams.

Stronger forward planning in primary care

Forward planning in primary health care teams is being encouraged by:

- the production of comprehensive health strategies by health authorities

- the improved integration of primary health care teams leading to a single plan for GPs, practice staff and community nurses

- the need for forward planning in fundholding.

Forward planning is being actively encouraged by health authorities and many departments of public health are working with primary health care teams to plan for practice populations using local epidemiological data. This work covers planning for the services primary health care teams provide themselves, and planning for hospital services purchased by health authorities to support the primary health care teams.

Increased accountability for GP fundholders

The responsibility for managing and monitoring GP fundholding has gradually passed from regional health authorities to FHSAs to health authorities. At the same time, the accountability of GP fundholders has been clarified nationally.

Fundholders' budgets are subtracted from the allocation of money to district health authorities. Use of this money was then monitored by the FHSA. Merger means that the source of fundholders' budgets (the DHA) and the agency responsible for monitoring those budgets (the FHSA) are now the same organization. This tends to increase the scrutiny of the financial aspects of fundholding and has led to unease amongst fundholders who are concerned that the financial pressures on district health authorities will now be passed on to fundholders, and that control and monitoring mechanisms will become increasingly stringent.

GP fundholders as partners in planning

It is not possible to produce a single health strategy without involving local GP fundholders as partners in planning. This gives GP fundholders the opportunity to influence the DHA's historical role more than ever before. The potential is clearly there for co-operative purchasing of community and hospital services under the auspices of a shared health strategy. In many parts of the country this potential has yet to be realized.

Barriers, limitations and challenges to the new health authorities

If the new health authorities are to achieve their full potential they must overcome a complex range of barriers and difficulties. The following section uses current experience to predict the main problems that will need to be faced.

Central control at national level by the Department of Health, NHS Executive and NHS Executive Regional Offices is likely to continue to increase, particularly in areas such as performance targets (e.g. meeting Patient's Charter standards). At the same time it is likely that devolution of politically sensitive decision-making to health authorities will continue (e.g. decisions about rationing services).

Maintaining local 'healthy partnerships' will continue to be difficult because of conflicting national policy. For example, relations with social services are likely to be strained because the NHS is free at the point of delivery but social care is means-tested. Lines drawn locally between health and social care will therefore continue to determine who has to sell their house to fund care and who does not.

Financial shortages will continue to affect the UK health care system for the foreseeable future. This will continue to make work on priorities and rationing a key (but fraught and unpopular) task of the new health authorities. Working with the public, practitioners and trusts to develop a real understanding of the financial position will be a major task. This task is made more difficult by the increasingly expensive new treatments made possible by technological advances and new drugs.

Developing clinical consensus, as success in working across primary and secondary care depends on making decisions backed by the majority of local clinicians. The new health authorities will need to understand and work with the formal and informal labyrinthine networks in both primary and secondary care if this is to be achieved.

Personnel 'crises', as applications for GP, consultant, junior doctor and nursing posts are declining in some specialties and in some areas of the country. This could be the start of a trend which indicates that the modern NHS is a less attractive career option than previously. Reasons for this are complex and may be influenced by decreasing public regard for health care workers and a perceived change in the underlying ethic of the NHS, away from 'caring' towards 'business'. There may also be a perception among GPs and consultants that their traditional professional autonomy is being gradually eroded, resulting in a corresponding decline in job satisfaction. It is very difficult to predict the strength of these trends, but foresighted purchasers and providers will be monitoring the situation very carefully and considering changes such as different skill mix patterns and task sharing.

Summary of implications of the reorganized NHS for general practitioners

1   Traditional 'pay and ration' functions of FHSAs should be unaffected.

2   Both fundholders and non-fundholders will be far more involved in health authority purchasing decisions (i.e. consulted much more about purchasing from hospitals and purchasing from community services).

3   Links with LMCs will remain crucial for negotiating with practitioners over the fine detail of their 'provider' role under the 'red book'.

4   Allocations of budgets to fundholders are likely to be more tightly controlled, as is the monitoring of fundholding.

5   Primary health care teams have the opportunity to become more united: GPs and practice staff will have opportunities to work more closely with health visitors and district nurses. Changes to traditional work patterns may help primary health care teams to offer a wider range of treatments.

6   Forward planning in primary health care teams will be strengthened, taking into account the needs of the practice population. Collaboration between GPs and departments of public health will increase to assist planning in primary care.

7   a) The consequences of GPs' actions (e.g. decision to refer, decision to prescribe etc.) will become more apparent, and will be scrutinized more closely.

    b) The consequences of consultants' decisions on primary care (e.g. change in prescribing recommendations, earlier discharge etc.) will be scrutinized more closely.

8   Trends towards increasing monitoring and quality control over GPs' actions will continue.

9 There is unlikely to be a diminution in the GPs' perception that they are working in an increasingly managed NHS.

10 With the abolition of regional health authorities, GPs will feel one step closer to increasing centralized direction of the whole NHS from the Department of Health and NHS Executive.

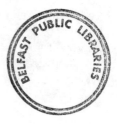

Index